THE SYSTEM OF HEALING USED BY THE
# FILIPINO ESPIRITISTAS

# THE SYSTEM OF HEALING USED BY THE FILIPINO ESPIRITISTAS

## Dr. Scott M. Taubold Ph.D.

Copyright © 2025 by Dr. Scott M. Taubold Ph.D.

All rights reserved. No part of this publication may be reproduced, distributed, or transmitted in any form or by any means, including photocopying, recording, or other electronic or mechanical methods, without the prior written permission of the copyright owner and the publisher, except in the case of brief quotations embodied in critical reviews and certain other noncommercial uses permitted by copyright law. For permission requests, write to the publisher, addressed "Attention: Permissions Coordinator," at the address below.

**CITIOFBOOKS, INC.**
3736 Eubank NE Suite A1
Albuquerque, NM 87111-3579
*www.citiofbooks.com*
Hotline:        1 (877) 389-2759
Fax:            1 (505) 930-7244

Ordering Information:
Quantity sales. Special discounts are available on quantity purchases by corporations, associations, and others. For details, contact the publisher at the address above.

Printed in the United States of America.

ISBN-13:    Softcover    979-8-89391-992-9
            eBook        979-8-89391-993-6

Library of Congress Control Number:

# THE SYSTEM OF HEALING USED BY THE FILIPINO ESPIRITISTAS: AN ARCHIVAL STUDY

Scott Matthew Taubold

Saybrook Graduate School and Research Center

The purpose of this dissertation was to describe the system of healing used by the Union of Espiritistas of the Philippines as perceived by the espiritistas themselves (in accordance with the National Institutes of Health Office of Alternative Medicine standards), from their own cultural context, not from the view of the parapsychological investigators, psychologists, medical doctors, alternative practitioners, and laypersons that have provided most of the existing information on Filipino healing practices.

The roles of indigenous healers were presented by prominent theorists, placing the practices of mediumship and psychic surgery into perspective as indigenous healing phenomena. The essential principles and common factors in healing as described in other systems of healing models were also presented. Following this description of the Filipino espiritistas' indigenous healing system, while incorporating these essential elements of healing (according to the prominent systems of healing theorists), this author's conclusion is that more research of indigenous healing practices in the Philippines is vital to a better understanding of the role of human consciousness in illness and healing experiences.

The research question was: What is the system of healing used by the Filipino Espiritistas? The study concentrates on descriptions of the

Filipino espiritistas' system of healing in accordance with the parameters for a healing system presented in a journal article in *Alternative Therapies in Health and Medicine,* "Defining and Describing Complementary and Alternative Medicine" by O'Connor et al. (1997). Archival data were utilized in gathering the necessary information to develop a description of the Filipino espiritistas' system of healing, and it was determined that the description meets the parameters of a system of healing as presented by O'Connor et al. to the U. S. National Institutes of Health Office of Alternative Medicine (NIHOAM).

# ACKNOWLEDGMENTS

I wish to express my gratitude to those who assisted in this study. My thanks to the members of my dissertation committee Stanley Krippner, Jeanne Achterberg, and Ruth-Inge Heinze-for their continuous guidance. Appreciation goes out to Harvey Martin, who provided more information on the Filipino espiritistas than any other single author; Emilio Laporga, who facilitated my personal experience at the hands of a former member of the Union of Espiritistas of the Philippines; my wife, Dolores Taubold, and her family-Pedro Baronda, Al Baronda, and Nenette Renshaw-who introduced me to tambalans in Cebu and acted as interpreters; and Virginia Thielen-Burns for her support through inspiration and manuscript preparation.

# TABLE OF CONTENTS

**I. INTRODUCTION** ..................................................................1

**II. LITERATURE REVIEW: INDIGENOUS HEALING PRACTICES** .................................................................15
    In the Philippines .................................................................15
    In the West .........................................................................22
        The 1950s and 1960s ...................................................22
        The 1970s .....................................................................26
        Other Reported Phenomena in the 1970s .............................36
        The 1980s .....................................................................38
        Anthropology in the 1980s .................................................40
        The 1990s: Complementary and Alternative Medicine ..........43

**III. ARCHIVAL DATA** ..............................................................50
    Personal Experience ............................................................50
    The Patients ......................................................................51
    The Healers ......................................................................53
    The Illnesses .....................................................................55
    The Healing Transactions ....................................................58
    Emilio Laporga ..................................................................63

**IV. METHODOLOGY** ..............................................................70
    Overview ..........................................................................70
        The Archival Method .......................................................72
        Advantages ....................................................................73
        Disadvantages ................................................................75
        The Inclusion of Personal Experience in the Archival Data ........77

## V. LITERATURE REVIEW: THE SYSTEMS OF HEALING MODELS .................................................................................. 79
Early Research .......................................................................... 79
The Systems of Healing Approach ............................................ 82
Kleinman: Patients and Healers in the Context of Culture ..................................................................................... 82
Frank and Frank: Persuasion and Healing ................................ 85
The Torrey Model: Witchdoctors and Psychiatrists .................. 87
Siegler and Osmond: Models of Madness and Medicine ......... 88
The Parameters for Complementary and Alternative Medicine ................................................................................... 90
Krippner and Remen: Systems of Healing ................................ 92
Applying the Archival Data to the Systems of Healing Models ...................................................................................... 93

## VI RESULTS ........................................................................ 95
The Parameters for Description of Complementary and Alternative Medicine ............................................................... 95
Lexicon .................................................................................... 95
What Are the Specialized Terms in the System? ...................... 95
How Are Common Health and Illness Terms Distinctively Defined by the System? .......................................................... 100
What Are the Terms Used to Identify Roles and People Within the System? ................................................................. 100
Taxonomy .............................................................................. 101
What Classes of Health and Illness or Disease Does the System Recognize and Address? ............................................ 101
What Causes for Illness Does the System Recognize? ........... 102
How Important Is It to Identify and Address Ultimate, as Opposed to Proximate, Causes of Illness? ............................. 103

Epistemology .................................................................104
Is There a Canonical Body of Knowledge?............................104
How Do the Origins and Social History of the System
Relate to Current Theories and Practices?..............................105
What Are the Internal Disputes and Variables of the
System?...................................................................................107
How Does the System Respond to Novel Input?...................108
Theories (Links to Taxonomy and Epistemology) ................109
What Are Important Human Systems, Their Mechanisms
Action, and Their Interconnections Understood to Be?........109
How Are the Symptoms Interpreted Within the System,
Generally and Specifically? ....................................................112
What Is the Relationship of Preventative and Therapeutic Actions
to Illness and Prevention or Melioration of Illness? .............112
What Is the Role of Patients' Beliefs or Expectations of
Practitioners' Intent? .............................................................113
Goals for Interventions .........................................................114
What Are the Primary Goals of the System?........................114
Outcome Measures ...............................................................114
What Constitutes a Successful Intervention?........................114
How Are Successful Interventions Evaluated?......................115
How Are the Successes and Failures of Treatments and
Practitioners Explained? .......................................................115
Social Organization...............................................................116
What Are the Prevalence and Distribution of This
System? ..................................................................................116
Who Uses the System or to Whom Is It Particularly
Accessible? .............................................................................117
What Is the System's Referral Network? ..............................117
Are There Specialist Practitioners? ........................................117

What Kinds of Specialists Are There? ...................................118
What Are the Usual Therapeutic Practice Sites?.....................119
What Are the System's Internal and External Legitimization and Oversight Structures? ..............................................................119
What Therapeutic Measures Are Undertaken at Home or Elsewhere, on One's Own or With the Aid of Family Members? ...............................................................................120
How Are Practitioners Compensated? ...................................120
How Does the System Interact With Other CAM Systems?................................................................................121
Specific Activities and Materia Medica ..................................121
What Do Practitioners Do?....................................................121
What Is the Specific Materia Medica? ....................................122
What Are the Classes and Purposes of Interventions?............122
Responsibilities ......................................................................123
What Are the Responsibilities of Practitioners? .....................123
What Are the Responsibilities of Patients or Clients? ............124
What Are the Responsibilities of Family or Community Members? ...............................................................................125
Are There Consensual Ethical Norms? ..................................125
Scope .....................................................................................126
How Extensive, Varied, or Specialized Are the System's Applications? ..........................................................................126
Analysis of Benefits and Barriers ...........................................126
What Are the Risks and Costs of the System From the Insider's Perspective?............................................................................126
Accommodation and Views of Suffering and Death..............126
How Does the System View Suffering and Death? ................126
Comparison and Interaction With Dominant System...........127
What Does the System Provide for Healing and for Coping

With Illness That the Dominant System Does Not Provide? ..........127
How Does This System View Interaction With the Dominant System? ..........128

## VII. MEDIUMSHIP AND PSYCHIC SURGERY AS INDIGENOUS HEALING PHENOMENA ..........131
Other Theoretical Perspectives ..........131
Winkelman's Schema ..........131
Hansen's Trickster Character Type ..........136
Walsh and Shamanic Trickery ..........143

## VIII. DISCUSSION ..........141
Martin: The Secret Teachings of the Espiritistas ..........141
Kleinman's Proposal ..........143
Frank and Frank's Contention ..........144
The Torrey Model ..........145

## IX. LIMITATIONS AND ISSUES ..........146
Brody and Brody's Model ..........147
Kleinman's Treatment Approach ..........148
Additional Delimitations ..........149

## X. SUMMARY AND CONCLUSIONS ..........151

## REFERENCES ..........161

## APPENDIX A PARAMETERS FOR DESCRIPTION OF COMPLEMENTARY AND ALTERNATIVE MEDICINE ..........165

PPENDIX B SSENTIAL HEALING PRINCIPLES AND COMMON FACTORS IN HEALING ..........................................167

APPENDIX C KLEINMAN'S INTERVIEW QUESTIONS.......168

APPENDIX D GLOSSARY DEFINITION OF TERMS, ABBREVIATIONS, AND CONVENTIONS ..............................169

ABOUT THE AUTHOR..........................................................180

# I. INTRODUCTION

The practice of so-called *psychic surgery* in the Philippines has fascinated many Westerners since the first accounts by observers reached the outside world in the late 1950s. The practice of psychic surgery by Filipino *espiritistas* (faith healers who claim to communicate with discarnate entities), a technique of purportedly entering the human body with bare hands and without the use of anesthetics, defies the laws of medical science as they are currently understood. Serious study of psychic surgery has been neglected by mainstream academic and scientific communities, simply because the phenomenon lies far outside the generally accepted concepts and applications of allopathic medicine, the dominant form of medicine practiced in the West and in other industrialized cultures. Psychic surgeons are under constant scrutiny because people often cannot believe their own eyes when observing the phenomena and assume the practitioners are merely master magicians utilizing sleight-of-hand.

In the West, this practice would commonly constitute fraud since the medical establishment does not recognize the use of therapeutic sleight-of-hand, which, at best, is considered to evoke a placebo or expectation effect resulting in positive outcomes. In spite of significant results of placebo surgeries performed in the early 1950s by Henry Beecher and Leonard Cobb and associates (cited in Harrington, 1977, p. 22), prior to increased ethical restraints in the United States, this practice has largely been scoffed at or ignored. However, the data will show that over the past half century, many patients continue to report remarkable recoveries at the hands of the psychic surgeons in the Philippines (Krippner, 1976; Krippner & Villoldo, 1976; Licauco,

1977,1992,1999; Martin, 1998, 1999; McDowall, 1998; Sherman, 1966; Sladek, 1976; Stelter, 1976; Valentine, 1973).

The earliest accounts of psychic surgery were published by curiosity-seeking laypersons in search of "fantastic and unusual" phenomena in Asia (Ormond & McGill, 1959). These early writings were followed in subsequent decades by publications that included speculations and theories by parapsychologists on this phenomenon and how it should be explained within academic and scientific communities. The data presented here have been compiled from popular books and scholarly articles written by parapsychologists, psychical researchers, anthropologists, and physicians, as well as practitioners of so-called New Age healing techniques and other professionals using complementary and alternative healing systems.

The research on psychic surgery is troublesome for several reasons that involve conceptual problems of the application of either parapsychological concepts or mainstream scientific methods to a spiritually based practice. Theories of the psychokinetic displays of alleged healers include materialization, dematerialization, and teleportation, as well as esoteric speculations about energy transference. It is debatable whether the technology exists to test these theories put forth by psychical researchers such as Meek (1987), Stelter (1976), parapsychologist Krippner (1976), and others, regarding how the psychic surgeons are affecting people's health and illness.

> We must remind ourselves that to this day we do not possess any scientific tool-any detector-that can furnish us with direct proof of psychic energies or thought. The measure of electrical brain waves (EEG) in no way directly establishes thoughts and feelings, as laymen believe; it may indicate nothing more than secondary action. (Stelter, 1976, p. 215)

The explanations that have been applied to the practice of psychic surgery range from the use of therapeutic sleight-of-hand producing a placebo effect (Krippner, 1976; Martin, 1998), or, on the other hand, to actual physical manipulations taking place through the spiritual body

(Lampis, 1999), the hypothetical bioplasmic body (Sherman, 1966; Valentine, 1973), or in the so-called fourth dimension (Ormond & McGill, 1959).

"Proponents point to controlled studies showing that humans are capable of both extrasensory perception (ESP) and of exerting psychokinetic (mind over matter) effects on objects and organisms" (Walsh, 1990, pp. 194-95). However, research outcomes based on scientific methods have generally been limited. An inclusive study will recognize that the practice of psychic surgery requires further research in the emerging field of complementary and alternative medicine, beginning with an accurate description of the Filipino espiritistas' system of healing.

## Purpose of the Study

The purpose of this study was to apply the body of historical archival data, combined with this author's firsthand experience, to the specific descriptive parameters for an alternative system of healing in order to produce a thorough and accurate description of the system of healing commonly referred to as psychic surgery. The descriptive parameters for complementary and alternative healing systems were published by O'Connor et al. (1997).

The U. S. National Institutes of Health Office of Alternative Medicine (later renamed National Institutes of Health National Center for Complementary and Alternative Medicine) commissioned a panel to develop parameters to define and describe complementary and alternative medicine. The Center's parameters were utilized in this study to describe the Filipino espiritistas' healing system. By fully describing the system of healing used by the Union of Espiritistas of the Philippines, a better understanding of their practices can be provided and may promote more effective research in the area of indigenous healing systems.

This study attempted to provide a description of the Filipino espiritistas' system of healing. O'Connor et al. (1997) defined a description of alternative healing systems as:

1) Discourse intended to give a mental image of something experienced.
2) Must derive from observation or experience.
3) When applied to a class of phenomena, may yield an aggregate set of features, all of which need not apply to each particularmember of the class. (p. 50)

Following an exhaustive literature search, and a review of this author's personal experience in the Philippines, a comprehensive description was made of the system of healing and practices of the Filipino psychic surgeons according to the parameters presented by O'Connor et al. (1997) in "Defining and Describing Complementary and Alternative Medicine," as they appeared in a journal article in *Alternative Therapies in Health and Medicine* (see Appendix A).

For the purposes of this study, it is assumed that information pertaining to the Filipino espiritistas was reliable if the information was consistent with other data gathered from documented eyewitness accounts, interviews, participant observations, and, most importantly, the espiritistas themselves. Data that were (a) congruent with the espiritistas' worldview, (b) fit the parameters for an alternative system of healing according to O'Connor et al. (1997), and (c) considered unique to the conditions they were intended to define have been utilized in the description to maximize descriptive validity.

## Statement of the Problem

Most of the inquiries into the phenomenon of psychic surgery in the Philippines have been conducted within the narrow frameworks either of a Western scientific worldview or of psychic research. Many researchers have focused only on attempts to determine if the psychic surgeons were actually entering the body wall and performing a real surgical procedure, or if they were simply masters of sleight-of-hand and practicing the art of deception (Krippner, 1976; Martin, 1998).

The faith healing methods of the espiritistas evolved from ancient healing traditions of Southeast Asia (Licauco, 1999; Martin, 1998; Singer, 1990), which are unfamiliar to modern Western societies; hence, conceptual barriers exist between indigenous folk healing practices and the practices of modern medicine. These barriers have contributed greatly to theoretical flaws and misconceptions in much of the research of psychic surgery. Few follow-up studies have been attempted that document the outcomes of patients' individual healing experiences.

Licauco (1999) reports, "I have seen cases of cysts, abscessed teeth, tumors, adenoma, multiple sclerosis, spinal deformity, leukemia, organic paralysis, and others that were cured by our healers" (p. 181). Although there have been numerous reports of positive outcomes from the patients, little comprehensive research has been performed that includes an understanding of the worldview of the practitioners and their system of healing. No other possibilities have been considered, nor has a culturally sensitive approach been used. Researchers have largely ignored statements made by the espiritistas about how they perceive themselves and their practices within their own spiritual belief system.

Psychic surgery, whatever its dynamics, exemplifies the complexity of the healing capacity of human beings and, therefore, deserves the attention of medical science, humanistic psychology, and related disciplines and warrants further research. Improved research may be conducted by recognizing and transcending previously limited models and by utilizing a systems of healing approach to broaden the possibilities of novel outcomes.

Allopathic medicine is the accepted healing system in the West and in industrialized nations. In recent decades, an explosion of interest in complementary and alternative medicine has resulted in the development of new models within which to research such healing systems (Pelletier, 2000). Many alternative healing systems have ancient historical roots. Indigenous healing systems require culturally sensitive research from psychological, anthropological, and ethnographic perspectives. The practical applications of these healing systems often require an examination of the role of human consciousness in illness and healing experiences.

Harvey Martin, a member of The Church of the Living Truth and a chiropractor, is perhaps the most learned Westerner regarding psychic surgery in the Philippines. Martin spent 8 years observing, filming, and participating in mediumship training within the Healers' Circle, a group of healers separate from the Union of Espiritistas of the Philippines. He has spent more than 10 years in his research of psychic surgery, became an ordained minister of the Healers' Circle, and was elected regional vice president for the United States.

Martin (1999) comments on the debunking of psychic surgery in the Philippines that took place during the 1970s:

> The publicity surrounding psychic surgery had drawn a number of people from around the world that saw themselves as public servants, boldly blowing the whistle on medical fraud. To these skeptics, psychic surgery was a brazen hoax with no redeeming value. As I came to know these people, flaws in their thinking became apparent. The most obvious was their total dismissal of the many dramatic, often miraculous, cures that were taking place. While working at Alex's [Orbito] healing center, I saw hundreds of people come from around the world with all sorts of ailments and leave cured. I began to wonder why the debunkers were choosing to ignore the obvious success of the psychic surgeons. (p. 3)

A good example of the ignorance and misunderstanding of this particular alternative healing method is "the case against psychic surgery," presented in *The Realms of Healing* (Krippner & Villoldo, 1976, p. 1). On February 28, 1975, Judge Daniel H. Hanscom (1975), an administrative law judge, acting in response to an action instigated by the Federal Trade Commission, declared psychic surgery a fraudulent practice and ordered several travel agencies to stop promoting "psychic healing" trips to the Philippines. The entire transcript of the court hearings covered 2,388 pages of both pro and con testimonies from patients and observers who had experienced Filipino faith healing.

Some witnesses testified that the tissue samples removed from their bodies were laboratory tested, and determinations were made that the tissues were nonhuman. This alone convinced the judge that the psychic surgeons were utilizing sleight-of-hand. Other individuals claimed that the tissue samples tested were genuine these reports were ignored. Numerous claims have been made both for and against the authenticity of tissue samples provided for testing by psychic surgeons and their patients (Sherman, 1966; Valentine, 1973; Watson, 1974). "Hanscom's decision ran only seventy-five pages and completely ignored all testimonies supportive of the Filipino healers' claims" (Krippner & Villoldo, 1976, p. 6).

Judge Hanscom declared that psychic surgery was fakery, "simply phony." However, from the earliest accounts to the present there have been numerous reports of fraud and deception by Filipino psychic surgeons, as well as reports of anomalous healings by satisfied patients, who frequently returned for further treatment by these practitioners.

There is a critical point regarding the research of psychic surgery in the Philippines made by Krippner (1976), Martin (1998, 1999, personal communication, January 18, 2002), and others. Any investigation of alternative healing, to be intellectually honest and open-minded, needs to address the question of whether psi (psychic phenomena) may play some role.

> If you permit yourself to be influenced by a few reports of fakers and quacks, you might be disposed to dismiss all purported faith and spirit healings as not warranting the time and expense of investigation. There is obviously not space in this or ten other books to detail the vast pro and con material. (Sherman, 1966, p. 159)

As William James (cited in Walsh, 1990) said, "There is no source of deception in the investigation of nature which can compare with a fixed belief that certain kinds of phenomena are impossible" (p. 195).

Krippner uses William James' analogy of the white crow to illustrate the danger of discontinuing certain types of research prematurely due to narrow thinking:

> William James, thefounderof American psychology, investigated several self-styled "psychics" and "mediums," noting that most of them were obviously fraudulent or engaging in self-deception. However, James wisely observed that one only has to see one white crow to prove that not all crows are black. (1976, pp. 10-11)

James' statement represents one of the basic premises upon which empirical research is based, demonstrates how inadvisable it is to jump to conclusions, and points out the advisability of keeping an open mind. Just because there are some fakers does not mean other practitioners are not genuine. Yet, this simple notion that not all things are equal is not taken into account when it comes to ideas so foreign to Westerners, such as a spirit-medium entering the human body with bare hands. Judge Hanscom and others did not allow for the possibility that some of the psychic surgeons may not have been practicing sleight-of-hand and that some were genuine white crows.

A second point to be made involves the oversimplification of possible research outcomes. Martin (1998) states:

> In the mid 1980s, virtually every researcher I met in the Philippines strictly limited the scope of their inquiries to the nature of the operation. Debate raged over two main issues: (1) Were psychic surgeons actually opening the body with their bare hands, or were they merely performing sleight-of-hand and (2) were the tissue and blood samples of animal or human origin? (p. 153)

Judge Hanscom, in the same manner as the early researchers, had not allowed for the possibility of healing through psychic surgery due to the power of faith, belief, placebo effect, social expectation, or other interaction effects. Nor did the judge consider alternative explanations for this phenomenon that reportedly promotes healing in afflicted individuals treated by the Filipino espiritistas.

Most accounts by Westerners did not consider the placebo effect as a possible explanation for the positive outcomes. Surprisingly, medical surgery, as a technique of intervention, is a treatment modality that is especially prone to the placebo effect (Vergano, 2000). Some of the highest percentages of positive outcomes from placebo effect are in relation to "placebo surgeries." Many of these studies were performed in the late 1950s (Harrington, 1977). Two controlled studies in the United States reported 68% and 91% improvement in patients who received placebo surgery for angina pectoris (Beecher, 1959). In his informative essay, "Unraveling the Enigma of Psychic Surgery," Martin (1999) states:

> In the late 1950s, several American doctors had concluded an experiment designed to determine the merits of surgical procedure for angina pectoris. In the experiment, three of five patients received the operation. The other two were merely placed under anesthesia and given a surface incision, which was then sutured. The five patients were monitored during their recovery from the operation. A significant percentage of the patients who had received placebo operation were cured. In 1961, Dr. Henry Beecher reviewed two double-blind studies of the placebo operations. These studies convincingly demonstrated that the actual operation produced no greater benefit than the placebo operation. (p. 2)

Martin (1998, 1999), Krippner (1976), and others perceived the placebo effect to be a viable explanation for at least some of the observed and reported positive healing outcomes of psychic surgery.

These are two main points that suggest the need for revision of the "rules of the game" in the research of psychic surgery (Krippner & Villoldo, 1976, p. 21). First, if it is determined that one surgeon utilized sleight-of-hand during one operation this does not indicate that all surgeons always utilize sleight-of-hand. Secondly, the use of therapeutic sleight-of-hand often promotes positive outcomes, as is customary with a placebo or expectation effect. The reality of the placebo effect as a medical concept is commonly accepted in the West. However, it is only addressed generally as a variable in medical research.

"In their haste to link psychic surgery to Western science, early researchers of psychic surgery largely ignored the cultural background of the phenomenon as it was understood by Filipinos" (Martin, 1998, p. 152). Like Judge Hanscom, researchers such as Nolen (1974), who detected occurrences of sleight-of-hand, wrote off the entire practice as fraudulent and discontinued any serious research of the phenomena, a closed case of black and white (either/or) thinking. Investigators did not take into account the "surgeons" who were performing similar indigenous healing practices that their local *mananambal* (Filipino magico-religious healers of the shamanistic tradition) had been practicing effectively for thousands of years.

Twenty-five years following the Judge's decision, a local Filipino researcher, Jaime Licauco (1999), responded to lingering questions regarding the viability of psychic surgery.

> There have been a significant number of cases considered incurable by ordinary medical science but which were indisputably proven to have been cured by faith healers in the Philippines e.g.-cases of terminal cancer, leukemia, paralysis, etc. There have also been, on the other hand, many cases of spectacular failures. Obviously the question of effectiveness is one area that requires much further study and documentation before a definite answer can be arrived at. (p. 182)

Although researchers and promoters of psychic surgery have made several claims regarding percentages of positive outcomes, there is no hard data to prove its effectiveness. Hard data on the effectiveness of psychic surgery and other spiritually based healing systems are nearly nonexistent.

Early researchers lacked a cohesive paradigm by which to observe, evaluate, and understand the practice of psychic surgery; emerging "systems of healing" perspectives were as yet unavailable in the 1960s. Yet, the basic questions still remain. Is psychic surgery authentic, and is it effective? Some additional questions that require answers are: What exactly constitutes an effective outcome? What criteria should be used in making this determination? A decrease of symptoms, increase in physical health, emotional well-being, and spiritual growth are all possible positive outcomes that could result from psychic surgery.

These questions and suppositions exemplify the need for the use of systems of healing theoretical frameworks, such as the Parameters for Complementary and Alternative Medicine (O'Connor et al., 1997), within which to examine psychic surgery and other spiritually based alternative healing systems. More research is critical regarding the effectiveness of this healing system and other indigenous and spiritually based healing systems, apart from the biomedical model.

> The definition does not mention biomedicine or take biomedicine as a standard against which other healthcare activity and belief are to be measured A stringent effort was made throughout the [Office of Alternative Medicine] panel's deliberations to exclude bias and partisanship from its statements and recommendations. (pp. 52, 57)

The current investigation is an effort to present descriptive material as objectively as possible, based on both historical, archival data and primary sources. By drawing on these resources, a more comprehensive study of the espiritistas, faith healers, and psychic surgeons of the Philippines will place the research on new footing, inclusive of the healers' cultural context, while attempting to find a good fit between this system of healing and the parameters for alternative healing systems (O'Connor et al., 1997).

## Rationale

The attempt to describe indigenous healing systems with a new perspective, without the use of interpretations generated by the dominant biomedical system, appears to have gained some credibility. Dissatisfaction with the dominant research trends in science and medicine over the last several decades has resulted in the U. S. government's response through the formation of the National Institutes of Health Office of Alternative Medicine (NIHOAM). "The NIHOAM encompasses all health systems, modalities, and practices and their accompanying theories and beliefs, other than those intrinsic to the politically dominant health system of a particular society or culture in a given historical period" (O'Connor et al., 1997, p. 50).

This innovative approach to evaluating health systems is a much needed departure from research models of the past. The term *CAM* (complementary and alternative medicine) embraces numerous indigenous healing systems. Some of these systems have existed for many hundreds of years prior to the development of the current biomedical model. The primary focus at present is to discover and describe the beliefs and healing systems of the Filipino espiritistas as they correspond to the new modalities of alternative medicine.

Information on the healing systems of the Filipino espiritistas was obtained from an exhaustive literature search on the topic of psychic surgery and related Filipino indigenous healing practices. Included in the research are the earliest written accounts of psychic surgery published in the West, primary sources, direct accounts, cross-disciplinary literature published over the last half century, and personal participation. As a departure from previous research, O'Connor et al.'s (1997) parameters were chosen as a framework to apply historical and archival information from authors with varied backgrounds, to screen for personal bias, and to provide an alternative to the Western biomedical model.

> It is essential that scholars and researchers base descriptions of components and subsets of CAM on observation and inquiry and avoid introducing interpretations [e.g., what something really is or means or what is really happening] into descriptive material. Appropriate descriptions of CAM systems must be able to yield categories and representations that members of the system would themselves recognize as accurate and be able to verify. Interpretations are suitable research hypotheses or theoretical aspects of analysis and should be clearly identified as such and separated from descriptive elements in research proposals and reports. (O'Connor et al., 1997, p. 53)

The existing literature, interviews, and the recorded personal participation in psychic surgery provided the information necessary to describe. Cultural, contextual, and historical considerations have been accounted for, as much as possible, by applying the CAM parameters. Early accounts by curious Westerners offer only minimal information, but, they may be used collaboratively with more current information. The later writings reflect a more inclusive worldview, which allows for the validity of alternative healing systems.

Perspectives from the disciplines of psychology, anthropology, and/or parapsychology have benefited researchers who have spent time in the Philippines observing the espiritistas. Some investigators also participated in training and practice with the espiritistas. These more recent accounts are more esoteric and emphasize the espiritistas' spiritual belief system with less of an attempt to explain the phenomenon scientifically or according to parapsychological explanations. These perspectives provided the best fit with the descriptive parameters for complementary and alternative medicine.

## The Research Question

The research questions approached in this study were: What is the system of healing used by the Espiritistas? Does the Filipino espiritistas' system of healing (which includes so-called psychic surgery) meet the parameters for an alternative healing system as presented by O'Connor et al.? In the 1997 journal article, "Defining and Describing Complementary and Alternative Medicine," these parameters were presented as a new, comprehensive framework for the study of and emerging interest in alternative medical practices (see appendix A).

In posing the research question, I do not want to give the impression that there is a uniform, monolithic healing system. I am making generalizations for the purpose of simplicity. The Philippines is comprised of many diverse subcultural groups, each expressing some differences from the general system I am describing. Christianity was readily absorbed into indigenous Philippine culture after the Spanish conquered, then colonized, the Philippines more than 400 years ago. Approximately 90% of the Filipino population is Christian (Panopio, Cordero-MacDonald, & Raymundo, 1994, pp. 227-251). Filipino espiritistas commonly use the Christian-influenced aspects of the system described. The Christian concept of the Holy Spirit has become the main context within which the healers work. Individuals use some differences in their healing techniques, and their beliefs may slightly differ. The results of this study claim to be valid for the purposes of descriptive validity in accordance with the CAM expectations for a description of a system of healing (see Purpose of Study).

# II. LITERATURE REVIEW: INDIGENOUS HEALING PRACTICES

## In the Philippines

An extensive literature review was performed in Cebu City, but materials on indigenous healing practices were difficult to find. After visits to the Cebu City Public Library and networking with local contacts who had access to the large university libraries in Cebu City, it was determined that written information on indigenous healing practices on the island of Cebu was nearly nonexistent. There is a minimal amount of literature published by Filipinos themselves. Most of the literature that could be obtained was found in newspaper articles from the 1970s on the controversial topic of psychic surgery in the Northern Luzon region of the Philippines.

Westerners who spent time in the Philippines wrote most of the literature within the last half century, and this constituted most of the archival information. Most of these authors-psychical researchers, reporters, and laypersons-have worked outside the mainstream scientific and academic communities, as do the healers they have investigated. Additionally, several physicians contributed to the body of information.

The Philippines are made up of many diverse Southeast Asian cultures, but they have been greatly influenced by Western culture and Roman Catholicism. Obtaining information on the Filipinos' indigenous healing systems is extremely difficult, partially due to the historic power of the Roman Catholic Church and subsequent persecution of indigenous healing practitioners. There is also great diversity in worldview within the country's own native and immigrated peoples. Yet, the Philippines are the only Asian country where the majority of the people are currently of the Christian faith. The Spanish colonized the islands more than 400 years ago and maintained their control over the native people until about the end of the 19th century, at the time of the Spanish-American War.

There has been a lack of serious research performed regarding the indigenous shamanistic practices common to this part of the world. Many different alternative healing systems exist today in the Philippines worthy of closer examination. However, it is difficult to research these systems of healing for several reasons. Not only is archival data regarding pre-colonial healing practices largely unavailable, the people who engage in shamanistic healing remain outside the mainstream and are reluctant to share information about their healing methods, particularly with foreigners acting as participant-observers.

Ben E. Garcia (1985) refers to some forms of healing the Catholic Church does not endorse as congruent with Catholic beliefs, calling some practices "primitive" and "lower class." The Catholic Church has attempted to influence believers to refrain from utilizing the services of those practitioners they perceive as not adhering to standards set by their interpretation of the Holy Bible. The Catholic Church in the Philippines has attempted to establish ethical standards in regards to the healing practices of its members and does not acknowledge the use of therapeutic sleight-of-hand. Among the forbidden methods of healing are the practices of mediumship and psychic surgery.

The Catholic Archbishop of Cebu has endorsed several books on the topic of faith healing. Garcia (1985), an accomplished author and National Chairman of the Catholic Charismatic Healing Ministry of the Philippines, and Efren V. Ramirez (1995, 1996), a lawyer; law professor; and author of several political, religious, and law books, are two authors whose publications on faith healing are supported by Church officials. Catholic authorities specify which forms of faith healing the church endorses and which it does not. The Catholic Church has a narrow perspective regarding faith healing, and it maintains that spiritism and psychic surgery are the work of Satan, "the fallen power." Therefore, the Catholic Church strongly discourages its members from receiving services outside of a narrow range of approved faith healing modalities, prayer, and exorcism (Garcia, p. 29).

Garcia's (1985) book is advertised on the book jacket as "an expose of paranormal phenomena which abound in our midst and deceive millions of people around the globe." Garcia reveals information about *lahid* therapy in his book, *The Truth Behind Faith Healing*. According to Garcia, psychic surgery is an improved or advanced equivalent to primitive lahid therapy. Lahid therapy supposedly removes or extracts foreign bodies or particles embedded in the flesh or bloodstream allegedly caused by black magic, spells, or the machinations of evil forces. Lahid, according to occult tradition, is a counter- power strength mechanism, which dissolves or dismantles evil works that inflict diseases on victims.

A white linen pouch, which contains ground herb root particles, is massaged tenderly on the disease-inflicted area for approximately 20 to 40 minutes. Solid particles such as stones, broken glass, bones of fishes, and insects (whole or in parts) are common items extracted. Garcia contends that lahid therapy was an act of trickery and was a precursor to the practice of psychic surgery by Filipinos (p. 16).

*Tandock* therapy was practiced on the island of Mino, near the large island of Mindanao. Tandock therapy included the making of half-inch incisions over afflicted areas of the body while a type of scope is attached and "thick blood" is drained out of the patient (Garcia, 1985, p. 15). This breaking of the skin was not combined with the extraction of objects as in lahid therapy. Garcia suggests that increasing Western contact and the exposure to modern surgical methods may have influenced the traditional Filipino healers who began the practice of psychic surgery in the late 1950s. The opening of the body followed by the removal of tissues instead of rocks, leaves, and bugs has a great resemblance to the espiritistas' form of psychic surgery.

Jaime T. Licauco (1977), considered by some to be an authority on paranormal phenomena and Philippine mysticism today, has written *Healing Without Medicine*. Licauco's introduction states:

> When a long series of articles highly critical of faith healing appeared in the *Times Journal*, a Manila daily newspaper, late in 1976, the Filipino public's interest in the subject was once more aroused. I addressed mainly non-faith healers in my articles. I wanted to show that there are other forms of healing being practiced in the Philippines, aside from the much talked about and much publicized faith healing, involving the sensational psychic surgery. (pp. iv-v)

Licauco (1977) proposed a classification system of Filipino faith healers' methods: (a) *pranic* or magnetic healing, (b) psychic or mental healing, (c) spiritual healing, (d) mystical healing, and (e) divine healing (p. 7). Spiritual healing is the dominant form discussed by Licauco and is practiced in the Philippines by the espiritistas. He does not include sorcery as a classification. Licauco's classification system includes practices that are utilized in the Northern Philippines and are not specifically recognized in the South, in the Visayan Islands, and the island of Mindanao. The Philippine healers are not limited to any one of the classifications by method. Their methods are usually eclectic and often defy categories of classification. The espiritistas may utilize several different methods and combine the use of herbal medications from their extensive knowledge base as well. Licauco, who promotes these alternative forms of healing, reflects, "Whether the Philippine medical profession will take up the challenge offered by psychic healing remains to be seen" (p. vi).

Licauco (1999), also the author of *The Magicians of God: Faith Healers in the Philippines and Around the World*, begins his book with a foreword written by Alfred Stelter, a psychical researcher who visited the Philippines in the early 1970s (see Western literature review section). Licauco's book provides anecdotal material of his own personal experiences with most of the prominent Filipino psychic surgeons (espiritistas). He includes interviews containing information on many of the prominent psychic surgeons who have practiced in the Philippines. He begins with the first psychic surgeon to emerge from the Union of Espiritistas of the Philippines, Eleuterio Terte, in the late 1940s.

Licauco (1999) reports that Terte performed the first reported psychic surgery within the group of Kardec spiritist followers, The Union of Espiritistas Church. As the story is told, while Terte was performing magnetic healing on a patient, suddenly his patient's body started opening up. Allegedly, he was able to remove gallstones and infected tissue with only his bare hands. From that time on, he has continued this work known as psychic surgery.

According to his son, Terte became a magnetic healer in 1925 after two angelic children repeatedly appeared to him when he was seriously ill and, from them, he accepted his gift for healing. Terte fought as a guerilla leader against the Japanese during World War II. He was captured and imprisoned more than a dozen times, and he always sought the aid of the Holy Spirit when he suffered at the hands of his captors. Licauco reports he did not practice healing during the course of the war.

Terte believed his special personal characteristics and strong faith in the Holy Spirit had direct impact on his healing interventions. It is said that he would not accept payment for services and believed if he did accept payment, he would lose his ability to perform healing. Licauco (1999) testified in regard to Terte:

> Throughout his healing ministry [Terte] appears to have lived fully by that code of conduct set by Jesus Christ. I saw his humble living quarters in San Fabian, which consisted of nothing more than a wooden cot. His entire library consisted of about a dozen different versions or editions of the Holy Bible. (p. 3)

Terte passed away in May of 1979.

During the 1960s and the early 1970s, Antonio (Tony) Agpaoa became the most well-known psychic surgeon in the Philippines. He was also, perhaps, the most controversial. Agpaoa was born in 1939 in Rosales, Pangnasianan. According to Licauco, Agpaoa, as a young boy of 5, played with invisible playmates whom most locals believed to be nature spirits, which are believed to exist everywhere. On many occasions Agpaoa would suddenly appear high up in the top of the Caimito tree near his home. No one observed him climbing, but he would unexpectedly appear there high up in the tree. His healing powers began very early in his life. It was reported that, at age 10, he would stop other children's bleeding and close their wounds. It was said that no scars ever appeared. Agpaoa died in 1982, at the age of 42, after a severe stroke and a cerebral hemorrhage.

Following Terte and Agpaoa, Alex Orbito became a prominent psychic surgeon in the Philippines in the 1980s. Orbito was born in 1940, in a small town 150 kilometers northwest of Manila. His parents were among the founders of the spiritualist movement in the Philippines. The claims made by Licauco (1999) and others are as follows. At age 14, Orbito became aware of his healing powers. He had numerous dreams in which he was healing a multitude of persons with a Bible in his hand. One morning he met a crippled woman he had dreamed about the night before. She also had received a dream that he had healed her. He prayed and rubbed her legs with coconut oil for about 40 minutes, after which he told her to stand and walk; she did so for the first time in nearly 20 years.

Orbito claimed that he was not interested in pursuing healing as a profession. He saw that healers were underpaid and not appreciated in his community of Pangasinan. He moved to a more urban area and worked as a bus conductor, newsboy, and shoeshine boy. Twice Orbito became gravely ill, and twice he received a message from God to return to his home community and take up "his calling as a healer." Circumstances beyond coincidence led him back home, where he began his healing ministry. According to Licauco (1999), Orbito believes the hand of God guided him.

Licauco (1999) wrote two chapters in *The Magicians of God* regarding another prominent psychic surgeon, Jun Labo, who he refers to as one of the most controversial and colorful healers in the Philippines. Labo was born in Dagupan City in the Pangasinan province in the Philippines in 1934. His parents were members of The Union of Espiritistas Christiana de Filipinas. Like Orbito, Labo claims he initially did not want to be a healer. Joaquin Cunanan, the acting president of The Union of Espiritistas Christiana de Filipinas, encouraged him to develop his gift for healing. According to Licauco, Labo claims 75% to 80% effectiveness with his healing methods of magnetic healing and psychic surgery.

According to Licauco's (1999) book, Labo is a world traveler and has practiced psychic surgery in Australia, Belgium, Canada, Germany, Greece, Hong Kong, Japan, the Netherlands, Switzerland, and the United States. In the early 1980s, Alan Newman produced a film of Labo performing psychic surgery. The film was narrated by a popular American movie actor, Burt Lancaster.

Licauco (1999) devoted several chapters of his book to the psychic surgeon Emilio Laporga, who he referred to as "the healer who pulled my tooth without anesthesia" (p. 72). Licauco reported, "I found his method to be an exact copy of Blanche's" (p. 73) (see In the West literature review section). Laporga admitted having been, at one time, an assistant of Blanche's but denied that he learned the practice of psychic surgery from him, saying instead, "It is a gift." In March of 1989, Licauco and Laporga together attended the First International Conference on Paranormal Healing in Buenos Aires, Argentina, which drew international attention.

> All the difficulties I encountered in bringing Emilio Laporga to Argentina vanished at the thought that we were able to help so many suffering people halfway around the world and established lasting goodwill and affection for the Philippines in a faraway land. (p. 83)

Literature on indigenous healing systems was difficult to find on the island of Cebu. Licauco's (1992 & 1999) books were obtained from National Books, a modern book store chain. The public and university libraries yielded several newspaper articles from the 1970s, as well as another book by Licauco (1977). Garcia's (1985) and Ramirez's (1995, 1996) books were published by various Catholic parishes and were stamped with an official endorsement by the Archbishop of Cebu. The sources did reveal pertinent information, both from Filipinos who support and from Filipinos who do not support the espiritistas' belief system and the practice of psychic surgery in the Philippines.

# In the West

## The 1950s and 1960s

Most of the literature on psychic surgery has been published in America, Australia, and England, and some in Germany, Italy, and Japan. Most of these writings were in the form of popular books, exemplifying the lack of serious research from the scientific, medical, and academic communities. Research on spiritually based healing systems at that time was very limited, due to the lack of alternative methods of inquiry. The accounts of psychic surgery were written by a parapsychologist, journalists, anthropologists, both allopathic and alternative practitioners, and laypersons (Cagan, 1990; Krippner, 1976; Krippner & Villoldo, 1976; Maclaine, 1989; Martin, 1998;

McDowall, 1998; Meek, 1987; Ormond & McGill, 1959; Sherman, 1966; Sladek, 1976; Stelter, 1976; Valentine, 1973; Wright & Wright. 1974). Writings by Western authors present problems due to differences in worldviews and are fragmented among the various disciplines of biomedicine, psychology, parapsychology, anthropology, and the esoteric traditions.

The Western literature review begins with a very early publication, *Into the Strange Unknown,* written by two curiosity-seeking observers in search of "fantastic and unusual" phenomena in Asia, Ron Ormond and Ormond McGill (1959). Ron Ormond was a Hollywood motion picture and television producer and Ormond McGill was an author, lecturer, and naturalist. Both men were keen students of esoteric wisdom, comparative religions, and anthropology. In their early accounts of the phenomena, they referred to one espiritista whom they observed, Eleuterio Terte.

> Terte is president of the San Fabian chapter of the Union Espiritista Christiana de Filipinas, a group of occultists boasting 148 centers scattered throughout the island republic with more than one million members. The organization is largely a spiritist group, but unlike many other beliefs in the Far East, it has its basis in the Christian religion. The term utilized by the group, in translation means spiritist and departs from spiritualism as we know it in certain facets. (p. 21)

Ron Ormond filmed Terte while observing him perform psychic surgery. Ormond reported that the lens of his movie camera was barely inches away as Terte's fingers seemed to disappear into the abdomen of a pain-ridden Filipina. In an attempt to assess the use of sleight-of-hand, Ormond asked Terte, who was already shirtless, if he would move his operating table out of the hut and into better light for the purpose of their filming. "In the open sunlight, any props, tricks, or gadgets he might have had within the hut would not be present. Also, if his operations were dependent on sleight-of hand, it would be much more detectable" (Ormond & McGill, 1959,

p. 19). They described him as a "fourth dimensional surgeon" and described his techniques as "amazing operations." Ormond and McGill surmised, "That man's either working miracles or he's the greatest magician who ever lived" (p. 34). This early account was followed by speculations and theories by psychical researchers of how this phenomenon could be explained according to academic and scientific communities.

Henry Belk, a businessman with an interest in the paranormal, had commissioned Harold Sherman (1966) to research the Luzon healers. Belk had previously observed Arigo, perhaps the most famous pschyic surgeon in the world, in Brazil in 1963. He also commissioned John Fuller (1974) to write the book *Arigo: Surgeon of the Rusty Knife*. Belk later advertised in *Fate* magazine for copies of the 8-millimeter color film he had made, along with his booklet, *Bare Hand Psychic Surgery,* an account of his studies with Terte and Agpaoa. "The package was available for seventy-five dollars" (Christopher, 1975, p.53).

Harold Sherman (1966), a president and executive director of the ESP Research Associates Foundation and the author of *"Wonder" Healers of the Philippines,* presented several speculations on how psychic surgery worked. Sherman is responsible for coining the term "psychic surgery" (p. 5). Martin (1999) said of Sherman, "He inferred that the spiritual healing practices of the Filipinos were comparative in some way to the surgical procedures of Western medicine" (p.1).

> It is this area of what has been termed "psychic surgery," the alleged ability of some healers to perform major operations with their bare hands, to open and close physical bodies, usually leaving no scar, which has challenged our attention, our very concepts of what can and cannot be done. (Sherman, 1966, p. 5)

In Western cultures, rigid barriers between the hard sciences, parapsychology, and religion are frequently encountered. Filipinos who utilize indigenous healing systems have a very different worldview and are less concerned about conceptual differences.

An understanding of psychic surgery across disciplines is difficult, because the spiritual realm is not subject to the proclivities of modern science. A lack of understanding of the religious beliefs and spiritual practices of the espiritistas has misinformed investigators' attempts to define what they observed. These conceptual differences between parapsychology and the esoteric traditions exemplify some of the problems in approaches to the study of the Filipino espiritistas' system of healing.

While observing psychic surgery in the Philippines, Belk and Sherman had several conversations with Guillermo Tolentino, the acting Vice President of The Union of Espiritistas Christiana de Filipinas. Tolentino replied, "Our mission, with the guidance of the Holy Spirit, is preaching of the kingdom of God and the healing of all manner of sickness and disease" (cited in Sherman, 1966, p. 80).

Ulpiano B. Guiang, a spokesperson for the Filipino Espiritistas, made the following statement to Sherman:

> We, in the Philippines, observe the constant perfecting of mechanical inventions abroad, but we also observe that the world has not yet perfected medical science to the point where it can cure or prevent many diseases. This is perhaps why many of our people are still seeking cures from our faith and spirit healers and will keep on doing so for some time to come. (cited in Sherman, 1966, p. 201)

Many psychical researchers investigated the Filipino espiritistas in the late 1960s and early 1970s. Hiroshi Motoyama, Ph. D. was, perhaps, the first psychical researcher to investigate the phenomena of psychic surgery in the Philippines (in 1965) with the use of electronic instrumentation. In 1972, Motoyama became president of the International Association for Religion and Psychology. He made three trips to the Philippines to study the healers there. Motoyama brought some of the healers to his laboratory, The Institute of Religious Psychology, in Tokyo for study. As an inventor of electronic equipment for detecting and measuring so-called human energy fields, he applied his multi-disciplinary background to this research (Meek, 1987, p. 301).

> Dr. Motoyama attempted to test Tony [Agpaoa] initially at Tony's home in the Philippines. Dr. Motoyama's apparatus was ruined when Tony turned on his invisible *God* power. When his own machine failed, Dr. Motoyama made an appointment with Tony at the University of the Philippines Medical School to observe his brain wave reactions on the electroencephalograph. (Sherman, 1966, p. 224)

Sherman's book, which reported these extraordinary events, opened a floodgate of foreigners coming to the Philippines for healing, most with Agpaoa in mind.

## The 1970s

Tom Valentine (1973), a reporter, author, and senior articles editor for the National Features Syndicate, published a book, *Psychic Surgery: The Story of Antonio Agpaoa, Spiritualist Healer of the Philippines, and the Astounding Facts About Successful Surgery Without Instruments, Anesthesia, or Pain.* Valentine's book included a foreword by Sherman. These early writings focused on the well-known psychic surgeons Agpaoa and Terte. Valentine also compared the work of the Philippine psychic surgeons with Arigo, the Brazilian spiritist and psychic surgeon.

During the early 1970s, Agpaoa was the most prominent healer in the Philippines. A commoner, whose gift for healing had only been appreciated by local Filipinos, Agpaoa suddenly became an international sensation. He was an independent practitioner who did not belong to the Union of Espiritistas of the Philippines and did not exhibit the same Christian humility as did the other healers at this time. He was a businessman and had been accused of fraud on numerous occasions. Regarding Agpaoa, Valentine (1973) states, "For every story that alleges fraud, I can dig up two that claim he's a miracle worker" (p. 31).

Valentine (1973) also reported on Dr. Motoyama's use of EEG readings to verify the efficacy of psychic surgery. Motoyama had EEG readings taken on a 9-year-old epileptic boy, named Jeffery, one week prior to and during a psychic surgery performed by Ricardo Gonzales, then 1 week following, and again 2 weeks following the procedure. The EEG reading made 1 week after the surgery indicated considerable improvement.

> The reading taken after two weeks showed additional improvement, especially in the left temporalis, where apparent epileptic patterns had previously registered. Two months after the psychic operations on his brain the boy was able to attend school full time. His previously expressionless face became expressive and fully animated. (p. 125)

Dr. Motoyama documented a psychic surgery "under controlled conditions" (Valentine 1973, p. 122) performed by Juan Blanche, and then he conducted a laboratory analysis of the tissue in The Far Eastern University Hospital laboratory. David Deleon submitted the report on September 28, 1968. The tissue sample was taken from a lesion of the right scapula region and was determined to be either normal subcutaneous tissue or fragments of a benign lipoma, an epidermal fatty cyst.

Valentine's book also explained psychical researchers' views of these phenomena as the possible exchange of so-called psi energies. "The laying on of hands healing technique seems to be explained by the Russians [psychical researchers], but they have not accounted for the opening and closing of the body and the tissue removal demonstrated in psychic surgery" (1973, p. 132). Valentine's book included photographs of Jose Mercado and Patitayan Placido supposedly performing psychic surgeries. It was reported that Virgilio Gutierrez also performed psychic surgery in a way similar to Agpaoa. However, the controversy continues even until today. For example, according to George Nava True, II (2001), Placido was allegedly caught using cow organs during his psychic surgeries and was arrested for fraud in 1989 in Oregon. However, the practice of psychic surgery grew in popularity in the early 1970s.

> The Spiritists, organized into the Union of Espiritistas Christina de Filipinas, have 500 chapel-like healing centers in the islands. There are 24 'spiritual surgeons' who are recognized by the group, and stories of miracle cures are common in the Philippines, where faith healing by Spiritists flourishes. (Valentine, 1973, p. 43)

In an article titled, *Faith or Fake Healing*, Don Wright and Carol Wright (1974) proposed the notion that psychic surgery is performed both by the espiritistas who had received mediumship training, as well as by charlatans posing as genuine healers. The Wrights reported that their arrival to the Philippines "was filled with hope and expectation" (p. 72). Tolentino recommended they see Virgilio Gutierrez for their father's ailments. "Virgilio was able to define the condition and tell all about his previous treatments. He began his treatment with magnetic healing" (p. 72). He continued over the course of 17 days with various forms of treatment, which included psychic surgery.

Upon their return to the United States, the Wrights reported, "Dad was re-examined by the same doctors who had treated him originally, and he was found to be completely healed" (Wright & Wright, 1974, p.72). However, during their stay in the Philippines, the Wrights also encountered "fake" healers who had not developed "gifts" of mediumship, nor were they members of the Union of Espiritistas.

> These fake healers have grown in number as a result of the great number of foreign visitors who have come here looking for a miracle of healing (which many of them have found) ready to bestow great amounts of cash on their benefactors. (p. 73)

Many foreigners came to the Philippines seeking these supposedly genuine spirit-directed faith healers. The Wrights further stated, "Like the California gold rush," these fake healers had descended upon the hotels of tourist row. Some of the healers advised the naive patients to stay in the hotel rooms until the healing was complete, to eliminate any competition. "Fake healers, charlatans without any training in the healing arts, became commonplace when the opportunity arose to make easy money at the expense of gullible foreign tourists" (Wright & Wright, 1974, p. 74).

Fraudulent healers' practices decreased when the opportunities to take advantage of tourists in the urban areas diminished in the late 1970s. However, a great outpouring of severe criticism from the West emerged when psychic surgery became a news item, as seen in the writings of Nolen (1974) and True (2001). Many westerners traveled to the Philippines in search of miracle healings, yet accusations of fraud abounded. The practitioners continued, without making rational defenses for their healing practices. "All this would not happen if it were not for the reputation of genuine healers in the Philippines who have helped thousands of people" (Wright & Wright, 1974, p. 76). The

Wrights, after their healing experiences in the Philippines, promoted that "more research needs to be done" lest the Filipino espiritistas lose the opportunity to make "a tremendous contribution to mankind" (p. 74).

William A. Nolen, M.D. (1974) led the charge for the American medical establishment against the psychic surgeons in a book titled *Healing: A Doctor in Search of a Miracle*. He completed a 5-year surgical internship at New York's Belleview Hospital, which was the basis for his first book, *The Making of a Surgeon*. He was on the board of editors of the Minnesota state medical journal, and his articles appeared both in medical journals and leading American magazines. Nolen claimed to be objective and open-minded. He was probably as open-minded as most other physicians in the United States were in 1974 where alternative medicine was concerned. Much of Nolen's information was based on interviews, and it would be difficult to determine if Nolen provided accurate information, since he made use of pseudonyms.

Nolen reported that his strength as a participant-observer was due to his experience as a surgeon. "Surgery is my profession. I can watch operations with an objective critical eye" (1974, p. 210). He observed David Oligani performing an operation and commented:

> David's first fingers were visible from the first phalanges, from the knuckles up to the first joint; the last two phalanges were doubled up almost into a fist. Then the first phalanges were shoved up into the fleshy folds of the abdomen. Someone who had never seen an operation and who was eager to believe might be persuaded that his fingers were actually in the abdomen and the liquid we could see was blood. No one who has ever seen an operation would be misled for a moment. (p. 184)

Nolen reported that Joe Mercado, "one of the best psychic surgeons, one who never has to fake it," performed a "sham" operation on him (1974, p. 205). "I knew with certainty that Joe's hands hadn't been in my abdomen" (p. 205). As a surgeon, Nolen stated he knew with certainty that Mercado had not penetrated his abdomis muscles, two bands of muscles about half of an inch wide, which run from the ribcage to the pelvis. He reported tightening his muscles, and he could feel Mercado's hands on the outside of his skin on the outside of the rectus muscles. He further reported, "I could see as he began that he had some reddish-yellow object palmed in his right hand" (p. 204). After busying himself with some poking and tugging he pulled up a blob of reddish-yellow tissue (lumps of fat). "I'd have loved to grab that specimen, but Joe immediately threw it in a bucket behind him and an assistant doused it with alcohol and set it on fire" (p. 204).

Nolen also commented on other operations he had observed. He reported on an eye operation that Juan Flores had performed.

> Flores had simply palmed an animal eye, probably one he had removed from a dead dog. I knew damn well it wasn't Cunanan's eye. There was no way the optic nerve could stretch to allow the eye to come out like that. But when you see an operation-all that blood and gore-you suspend your critical faculties, you become believers. You'll notice they never take both hands off the body. They have to keep their hands on the body to sustain the illusion. (1974, p. 210)

Nolen admitted to being easily deceived by magicians in his past experience, which is not an asset for the careful observation necessary to describe these controversial practitioners. He made little attempt to explain his observations of Josephina Sison's psychic surgeries. Sison was considered by many to be an ethical and skilled psychic surgeon, one of the least likely to utilize sleight of-hand.

Nolen received the names of 53 people who had been treated by psychic surgeons in the Philippines, and, after his return to the United States, he chose 5 cases to review. Nolen had selected only those cases which supported his position and bias. The first case he chose to report on was a woman with cancer who had become quite frustrated with her conventional medical treatment. Nolen himself referred to her treatment as having been mismanaged. He reported that, following the poor treatment, she went to the Philippines seeking "quack cures" (1974, p. 249). The other cases mentioned by Nolen were filled with allegations that patients experienced prolonged illnesses and required increased extensive medical treatments as a result of time spent in the Philippines and their failed healing experiences at the hands of the Filipino healers. In one case, he reported that a woman returned home, had another gallbladder attack, and more gallstones were detected. The other cases mentioned were of cancerous tumors that increased in size, one tumor that had resulted in a fatality.

Nolen did not report that any psychic surgery might be genuine, nor did he report one positive outcome that could not have been accounted for as a psychosomatic ailment responding to spontaneous regression. He seemed to blame the healers for their patients' choices to seek alternatives to the biomedical model, which had apparently failed them in many cases. The other authors who documented their observations while in the Philippines in the 1970s reported their experiences quite differently from Nolen. Many authors seem more credible than Nolen, due to less bias in their reporting (Krippner, 1976; Sherman, 1966; Sladec, 1976; Stelter, 1976; Valentine, 1973; Watson, 1974).

However, Nolen (1974) made some comments that are congruent with systems of healing theories, such as his speculations on the qualities of healers.

> It is possible that "healers" by their machinations, their rituals, their sheer charisma, stimulate patients so that they heal more rapidly than they otherwise might; this is why doctors who have warm rapport with their patients seem to get better results than doctors who treat their patients briskly and impersonally." (p. 274)

Nolen also commented on the significance of the power of suggestion, particularly when augmented by the use of hypnotism.

However, he suggested that it is "most useful in emotional and not physical disturbances "(1974, p. 287). And in his conclusion he stated, "Nature does a lot more to heal the sick than we do–in fact much of the time patients heal themselves" (p. 307). After 2 years of research, Nolen had still been unable to find any "miracle workers" (p. 308).

Looking into the healing phenomena, becoming reacquainted with the interweaving and interdependency of the mind, the nervous system, and the body itself, I have become increasingly aware that all of healing is, in a very real sense of the word, miraculous. God has given us minds, the workings of which we have barely begun to comprehend, and using those minds, we have been able to find the answers to many of the puzzling disorders that afflict us." (p. 308)

Marti Sladek (1976), a journalist and reporter, wrote a book, *Two Weeks with the Psychic Surgeons,* based on her experiences in the Philippines in 1973. In this book, Sladek reported three kinds of healing observed in the Philippines: (a) magnetic healing; (b) spiritual healing; and (c) material healing, which allegedly involves the opening of the body (i.e., psychic surgery). She and her husband visited many of the prominent psychic surgeons at that time. Among them were Juan Blanche, Juanita Flores, Virgilio Gutierrez, Jose Mercado, Alex and Marcos Orbito, Patitayan Placido, and Josephina Sison. Sladek's perspective was that of a journalist, although she, her husband, and friends had made the trip to the Philippines for their own healing needs. She did not attempt to explain the phenomena, but deferred to speculations of psychical researcher George Meek for the final chapter of her book.

Because of adverse publicity in the international media, Sladek (1976) reports that she added some supportive information in her book for people, like herself and her husband, who had positive healing experiences in the Philippines. For example, in 1973, after treatment by Placido for cancerous thyroid, the patient returned home and gave tissue samples from the operation to a consulting pathologist for examination. The pathology report, in all its detail, as presented by Sladek (pp. 250-252), verifies that the tissues were indeed human and corresponded to the operation the patient had received. The pathologist was curious to follow up with the patient for information about the "unconventional surgery" (p. 252). However, he was unable to do the follow up study.

Alfred Stelter (1976) published a book called *Psi Healing*, which was originally written in German and translated by Ruth Hein. Stelter provided the most extensive account of the phenomenon of psychic surgery to that date. He had spent a significant amount of time in the Philippines filming and observing the espiritistas and participating in mediumship trainings. He included many testimonials regarding the authenticity of psychic surgery and addressed the issue of conflicting results of laboratory testing.

Laboratory testing has consistently provided conflicting results as to the authenticity of blood and tissue samples. For example, in 1971, a television crew arrived in the Philippines to film Agpaoa's healing work. The blood samples they obtained were taken away for analysis. 'The Institute of Forensic Medicine in Heidelberg determined that [some of] the samples of blood were human blood. Analysis of the samples we [the TV crew] had secretly taken gave uniformly negative results: not human blood!" (Stelter, 1976, p. 180). According to Stelter:

> Other American doctors have claimed that on examination, some of Agpaoa's blood and tissue samples turned out to be chicken blood and flesh. The rumor continues to circulate and be given wide credence. Agpaoa's reaction to the accusation was to stop giving away samples of blood and tissue. (p. 115)

Stelter (1976) also reported cases of successful treatment outcomes. A young boy who was congenitally blind in one eye was operated on by Agpaoa. After the procedure, he was able to see with this eye for the first time in his life. "The boy was tested to the extent possible in the Philippines, [and after he returned home] he was checked by an eye specialist who could not find any changes in the eye's organic state and could not explain how the child could see" (p. 209).

A woman, referred to as Frau J., traveled to the Philippines for a number of ailments. "Her blood count and spectrogram, evaluated by computer, as well as tissue tests indicated an advanced precancerous condition" (Stelter, 1976, p. 174). She received seven separate treatments from Agpaoa, and then she returned home. "Blood and tissue samples and computer-evaluated spectrographic blood analysis showed a decidedly positive change and she continued to improve" (p. 175).

After years of unsuccessful treatment for a benign tumor in the hip, a young boy went to the Philippines in 1966 for treatment by psychic surgery. Juan Blanche performed the operation on the boy, and, evidently, removed the entire mass. After returning to the United States, an X-ray was taken that revealed that the tumor was no longer there (Stelter, 1976, pp. 164-166).

Psychical researchers Alfred Stelter (1976) and George Meek (1987), parapsychologist Stanley Krippner (1976), and others visited the practicing Filipino espiritistas in the early 1970s. Stelter, Meek, and Krippner all speculated on the phenomena they observed in the Philippines. Their speculations on the espiritistas' practices involved alleged phenomena such as dematerialization, materialization, and teleportation. "Dematerialization-is the disappearance of temporarily or permanently organized substances in various degrees of solidification" (Meek, p. 61). Practitioner Josephina Sison exhibited this phenomenon of dematerialization. She is known for her technique as a psychic surgeon who supposedly pushes cotton balls (soaked in blessed oil) into the body wall, then pulls the blood soaked cotton balls back out, usually from another part of the body. Krippner (Krippner & Villoldo, 1976) reported his experience with this phenomenon:

> Sison pressed the wad of cotton, which measures about one inch by one half an inch into the right side of my body. Sison moved her hands to the left side of my abdomen. While I watched, the cotton appeared to vanish into the skin until only a small tuft remained. As Sison gave this a pat, it also disappeared. (p. 8)

Materialization, the second theoretical model, is the alleged appearance of "temporary, more or less organized substances in various degrees of solidification and possessing human, animal or mineral properties" (Meek, 1987, p. 61). Krippner continued to describe his experience with Sison, which may exemplify the materialization theory:

> As Sison brought her fingers to my side, a piece of cotton appeared to protrude from my skin. She began to pull it up and I could see that it was streaked with red. The cotton appeared to be sticking halfway out of my body. Then she finished removing the cotton and I could see traces of red fluid on either side of it- but no coconut oil. (Krippner & Villoldo,
> 1976, p. 8)

Meek (1987) elaborated on an example of alleged materialization:

> When Blanche treats a patient with a skin disease he sometimes seems to be pulling through the skin, spindle-like pieces of a yellow substance that looks like very small grass blades. However, the texture is more like a wax. I have seen this phenomenon many times under conditions where fraud is absolutely impossible. (p. 77)

Meek's (1987) explanation of the third theory, teleportation, which is supposedly accomplished by the teleportation of molecules. "When an object, either animate or inanimate, which after apparent penetration, through matter such as buildings, often arrives at the scene of action following a seemingly instantaneous transmission or teleportation from nearby, or from thousands of miles away" (p. 61). The teleportation theory is the most common explanation for materials extracted from patients who are perceived as witchcraft victims. The speculation regarding witchcraft victims is that when a hex has been placed on an individual, what occurs is the absorption of negative energy in the body. The claim is made that the surgeon does not know what form the negative energy will take when it is removed from the body as the surgeon operates. Rope, cassette tape, rocks, leaves, and so on are among the objects apparently removed from the bodies of witchcraft victims by psychic surgeons (Martin, 1998; Valentine, 1973).

# Other Reported Phenomena in the 1970s

Juan Blanche was a well-known psychic surgeon in the 1970s. He incorporated folk medicine techniques into his practice, such as the ancient art of cupping. In cupping, one creates a small incision, then lights a small piece of cotton soaked in alcohol and places a small glass cup over the incision. This seems to create a vacuum, which gently pulls blood or other bodily fluids out of the body through the incision. This author observed the technique of cupping used by Emilio Laporga in Cebu City in 2001 (see Archival Data section). Licauco reported that Laporga studied under Blanche and that their techniques were nearly identical.

In his practice, Blanche would sometimes grab the wrist of an observer, straighten out the forefinger, and then used that person's hand to make an "incision" on a patient from several feet away. The Sladeks (1976) observed Juanita Flores opening the body in this manner with "a slicing motion that appeared to be a combination of the slash technique of Blanche and the massaging techniques of Alex and Virgilio" (p. 202). Krippner (1976) observed Blanche use his finger to apparently open the body from a distance, a technique called "distance cutting" (Krippner & Villoldo, 1976):

> After folding his hands and uttering a silent prayer, Blanche indicated, by gesture, that I should extend the forefinger of my right hand. He then took my right hand and aimed my forefinger at the woman's back. He brought my finger to a point about six inches from the skin and just underneath the shoulder blade. Suddenly he made an abrupt motion with my forefinger, then released it. I noticed a slit on the women's skin in the exact area beneath my finger position. (pp. 206-211)

George Meek (1987) also observed this phenomenon:

> I take the point of view today that Blanche can under favorable conditions make the incision from a distance without touching the body of the patient. I think that it takes less effort for the healer to

produce an opening if his finger touches the patient, than when he does it from a distance. (p. 74)

A similar technique to Blanche's distance cutting is that of Jose Mercado's so-called spiritual injections, which patients stood in line to receive. Mercado supposedly injected the Holy Spirit from an invisible hypodermic needle, while standing a few feet away.

> Meek (1987) received several of Blanche's spiritual injections. The healer reaches into the air for an imaginary hypodermic needle, which he then places on the Bible, in order to "charge it." Then he aims it at the patient, moves a finger as if he were giving a shot, often without touching the body, and sometimes from a distance as much as one meter. At this treatment quite a bit of blood ran out of the entry point, and had to be wiped up several times with cotton before the bleeding could be stopped. (pp. 72-73)

Krippner (1976) also received a spiritual injection from Blanche.

> There was nothing in his hand, and nothing protruding from the tip of his finger, yet when he made a slight jerky motion with his hand, I felt a distinct needle jab. A tiny welt and a droplet of blood appeared on the spot. (p. 8)

Psychical researchers Stelter, Meek, and parapsychologist Krippner were among the most serious investigators who observed, reported, and promoted research of the phenomena of psychic surgery in the 1970s. These researchers made speculations from both paranormal and parapsychological perspectives.

Krippner (1976) observed psychic surgery in the Philippines and then wrote an article for *The Journal of Humanistic Psychology* and several chapters in a book (Krippner & Villoldo, 1976), *The Realms of Healing*. Krippner attempted to promote more serious research of the phenomenon of psychic surgery. He speculated early on that the healing which occurs is actually self-healing, inspired by the psychic surgeon's phenomenal displays, even though these effects may be attributed to legerdemain or therapeutic sleight-of-hand. Krippner also emphasized the need for an improved paradigm by which to research psychic surgery and other alternative healing modalities. Krippner and Remen (2000) later developed a "systems of healing" course, which was added to the curriculum at Saybrook Graduate School, San Francisco.

## The 1980s

In the 1980s, the United States witnessed both the rise and decline in the popularity of the New Age movement. During the two prior decades, a great surge of popular interest in the paranormal occurred, but was followed by a decided shift within the New Age and psychic subcultures.

The number of books published on paranormal topics dropped precipitously between 1980 and 1982. With the general shift away from psychism and toward the search for meaning, the books of Joseph Campbell became popular. There were new magazines, catering to that general trend. (Hansen, 2001, p. 204)

Many who had previously been interested in psychic matters shifted their attention to more spiritual concerns that might be characterized as asearch for meaning. This was subtly foreshadowed when California-based *Psychic* magazine changed its name to *New Realities* in 1977. Channeling came into vogue, but, unlike spiritualism, there was little emphasis on verifiable information or physical phenomena. Channelers made dire predictions of "earth changes" and gave general advice, but they offered no evidence of their claims (Hansen, 2001, p. 204).

Shirley Maclaine (1989), in her book *Going Within,* and Andrea Cagan (1990), author of *Awakening the Healer Within,* and others used Alex Orbito and his practice of psychic surgery as the focus of some of their writings. These books were written with a New Age "flair," which was apropos during this time. These authors provided their own personal anecdotal material and eyewitness accounts, but they lacked any scientific support to verify the information presented. The authors offered no explanation of these phenomena, but, rather, accepted the practices on faith, as was popular with the study of alternative health practices during the years of the New Age movement. Debunkers of psychic surgery were quick to point out some of the flaws made by New Age thinkers:

> Maclaine profited spiritually and financially with Orbito. She learned about a marvelous New Age art, and she garnered a chapter for her bestseller. Orbito profited as well: He gets about a hundred dollars a minute for his services, according to magician James Randi, who is the premier authority on pseudoscientific fraud. Thanks to Maclaine, Orbito presumably collected the hundred $100-1-minute-offerings in two days, and was able to return home to the Philippines with a large amount of cash and publicity. (True, 2001, p. 4)

This notion exemplifies one of the universal essential elements of healing, that of expectant faith (Frank, 1974). If the elite clientele did not pay a high price for their treatment, it is likely they would not place a high value on the treatment. The clientele's consciousness regarding materialism remains consistent with the essential element of expectant faith. The espiritistas explained to Martin (1998), "Materialistic patients failed to value things that they received for free, and that paying substantial amounts of money for spiritual healing services raised their expectations of receiving the best possible treatment" (p. 159). Their beliefs increased their chances of positive outcomes.

The New Age movement was transformative in the popularity of spiritual beliefs without the support of scientific explanation. This movement spurred the populartrend towards areas ofcomplementary and alternative medicine. As the New Age practitioners became interested in the psychic surgeons during the 1980s, the discipline of anthropology in the United States finally offered some journal articles regarding the practice of psychic surgery.

## Anthropology in the 1980s

Richard Lieban (1967), a longtime investigator of healing modalities in the Philippines, wrote the most comprehensive book on Filipino witchcraft and sorcery, *Cebuano Sorcery*. Lieban's articles did not focus on the practice of psychic surgery specifically, but, rather, emphasized the dynamics that take place between patient and healer.

Lieban (1981) published a journal article in *Culture, Medicine and Psychiatry* titled "Urban Philippine Healers and Their Contrasting Clienteles." He reported the results of a study of four indigenous healers and their patients in Cebu City. Only one of the four healers was a psychic surgeon, Emilio Laporga. In the conclusion section of Lieban's article, significant social and medical contrasts were discussed, as well as their implications, with respect to clients and their health care. In 1996, Lieban published "The Psychic Surgeon and the Schizophrenic Patient: Crisis in a Medicodrama" in the journal *Culture, Medicine and Psychiatry*, which reported on Laporga being confronted with a particularly challenging client, a psychotic patient who disrupted his healing sessions. The paper described an incident in which analyzed Laporga's response and how he modified his usual clinical practice to meet the demands of this difficult situation. Many informative dynamics were revealed between patient and healer (see Literature Review: The Systems of Healing Models). Lieban explains that Laporga was, in some ways, not typical of the other Cebu healers, being the only healer who did not come from the ethnolinguistic group around Cebu City. Rather, Laporga was from the Northern Luzon region, where the practice of psychic surgery flourished.

> Ben [Laporga] was the only one of the healers who was not a Cebuano, the ethnolinguistic group inhabiting the Bisayan area of the central Philippines where Cebu City is located. He had moved to Cebu City from the northern province of Pangasinan in Northern Luzon in 1974. (Lieban, 1981, p. 219)

Philip Singer (1990), an anthropologist, published a journal article titled "'Psychic Surgery': Close Observation of a Popular Healing Practice" in *Medical Anthropology Quarterly* This brief medical anthropology report included a discussion of the use of sleight-of-hand as a viable technique for healing. He was willing to consider the effectiveness of psychic surgery from perspectives other than the biomedical model and included placebo effect as a possible cause for positive outcomes. Singer acknowledged Belk and Sherman as "pioneers in the study of Filipino healers, who laid the groundwork for the researchers who followed them" (p. 449). In 1986, Reverend Philip S. Malicdan, a psychic surgeon from the Philippines, and his wife were visiting Belk for 2 months, at which time a demonstration of psychic surgery was planned by Singer.

The demonstration took place at Kettering Magnetics Laboratory at Oakland University in Rochester, Michigan. Malicdan "operated" on eight subjects who had been diagnosed with minor medical problems, such as hemorrhoids and varicose veins.

> Malicdan's wife was present and acted as his assistant during the demonstration. Consequently the demonstration was planned to focus on the alleged phenomenon itself-the act of opening the body barehanded and removing organic material, including blood and tissue, which can be analyzed for pathology. The questions were proposed, Is the body penetrated with bare hands? Are the tissues removed? Is the opening closed without a scar? (Singer, 1990, p. 444)

Singer contended that "the videotape record indicates beyond any doubt that sleight-of-hand was used to create the illusion of mysterious withdrawal of diseased tissue from within the patient" (1990, p. 447). The tissue samples supposedly extracted from the patients were in an advanced state of degeneration, which indicates they were not removed at the time of the purported psychic surgeries. 'The tissue specimens, furthermore, showed no relationship to the parts of the various patients' bodies from which they had allegedly been removed" (p. 447). Among the conclusions were that Mrs. Malicdan had transferred organic materials to Philip Malicdan by way of the wash basin (and other means) until the time they could be used in the Malicdans' acts of deception. "The question of healing was specifically not addressed, since almost any type of disease may respond to placebo treatment, including the common cold, hypertension, or multiple sclerosis" (pp. 443-444).

According to Singer (1990):

Psychic surgeons have made a vital transition from traditional shamanism (extraction from the body of leaves, seeds, worms, hair, etc.) to a simulacrum of Western scientific medicine (extraction of blood, tissue, tumors, organs) and from traditional shamanic concepts to Western religious concepts of the Holy Spirit and the saints. (p. 449)

In Singer's conclusion, he stated, "I suggest that anthropologists can study the phenomenon of psychic surgery from two different perspectives: (1) as cultural behavior and (2) as a biophysical phenomenon in and of itself" (1990, pp. 443-444).

## The 1990s: Complementary and Alternative Medicine

The literature written in the 1990s reflects a broader sense of the worldview of the healers themselves, rather than maintaining strictly Western perspectives. Many of the books published in the recent decade elaborate on the healers' worldviews. Donald McDowall (1998) and Harvey Martin (1998, 1999, 2000a, 2000b, 2002a), both practicing chiropractors, are proponents of complementary and alternative medicine, and their perspectives reflect many of the current CAM views. However, Martin (1998, 1999) elaborates more extensively on placebo effect, whereas McDowall does not speculate on any notions outside the perspective of the healers themselves. These more esoteric perspectives are congruent with guidelines for the CAM descriptive parameters and other systems of healing frameworks.

McDowall (1998), an Australian writer, presents the practice of psychic surgery as described from the perspective of the espiritistas themselves. In *Healing: Doorway to the Spiritual World*, McDowall describes his experiences with Jun Labo, renowned psychic healer of the Philippines, and provides photographs. McDowall subtitled his book: *"A Healer's Journey of Insights and Experiences in the Spiritual World of the Philippines with Photographs of God's Communication."* McDowall provides considerable information promoting the effectiveness of psychic surgery. He reveals Labo's perspective, with an emphasis on spiritual principles. Labo, who was a participant in a research project at a hospital in La Crosse, Wisconsin, stated:

> I was tested in America, from among 23 Philippines healers. I was the last one tested. All the specimens I took from the patients were tested. There was a panel of 40 American doctors. I was the only one to pass the test. That was why I was chosen to go to the hospital at La Crosse, Wisconsin. (cited in McDowall, 1998, p. 80)

Labo claims he was the only Filipino psychic surgeon who had ever been asked to work in a United States hospital. "While at La Crosse his work was carefully observed by the doctors at the hospital" (McDowall, 1998, p. 80). They tested the tissue cultures and blood samples that Labo had removed from his patients and found they were consistent with each patient. "Doctors could not explain how the healings took place but confirmed there were healings" (p. 80). After a review by the hospital board, it was determined his work at the hospital was "justifiable and accurate" (p. 80).

In addition to his experiences with Labo, McDowall (1998) also reports meeting the prominent psychic surgeon Emilio Laporga, who was on his way to a healing seminar in South America. They met at a hotel in Makati, near Manila, and exchanged stories and spoke of their mutual friend, Jaime Licauco. Laporga reported that, at 8 or 9 years of age, while participating in mediumship training, he was given the gift of healing from his spirit guide, Mary Magdalene, during a dream. His spiritual teacher helped him to interpret the dream. McDowall's book reports that Dr. Crisostomo C. Abbu, Medical Office V, Chief, Division of Environmental Services in Cebu City, along with Dr. Felimon Alberca, observed Laporga's healing techniques in 1990. The physicians stated that Laporga's healing techniques, which involved so-called psychokinetic phenomena, did not involve fraud; he used no anesthesia, no scalpel, or other instruments to open the body. There appeared to be little, if any, discomfort to the patient, no post-operative shock, and no history of infections reported (p. 185-186).

McDowall (1998) traveled to the Philippines between 1991 and 1995. He reports on his meditation experience with his spiritual teacher, Jun Labo. He stated that when Labo entered the healing room, he appeared to be changed while he prayed before the triangular mandala on the wall. His presence was felt to expand, and the physical man seemed to disappear as his body began to absorb spiritual energy. It was possible to feel the change in his energy. When he began performing psychic surgery, he changed into a larger-than-life-figure. The supreme being seemed to occupy his body. "He seems to be only aware of about 40 percent of what is going on around him. A spirit guide seems to take over during the healings," as he worked under the influence of this spirit guide (p. 100).

Labo told McDowall (1998) that when he stood in full trance and held out his hands, he could provide McDowall and the others present with the spiritual power that he was channeling from his spirit guide. He touched their outstretched hands for only a few seconds. When he had touched all of their hands, the spirit that allegedly possessed him then explained it would be leaving. "We were told we should use the grace we had been given wisely" (p. 110). Labo would sometimes fall when he came out of trance. His assistants would usually catch him and help him to recover. McDowall observed Labo closely when he came out of trance. He seemed very cold and would have to warm up afterward. "I assumed there was a strong parasympathetic action within his body during trance. Probably most of the blood and circulation goes to the central nervous system and his brain" (p. 125).

McDowall (1998) elaborated on his experience in mediumship training under Labo. When Labo seemed pleased that the training was progressing, he told him he would test him the next day to determine if the spiritual power was coming through him during the healings. "I resolved to continue to pray and to build my meditation skills to become more receptive and better at focusing on this energy" (p. 35). Labo told him he would get stronger. Labo advised him to drink water frequently, because meditation often makes one thirsty and hungry as the parasympathetic nerve response will produce mild dehydration (p. 135).

McDowall (1998) made no attempt to explain why psychic surgery works, but he provided numerous accounts of its effectiveness and included many documented testimonies of satisfied patients. He did not limit his examples to physical cures. His success stories included healings of patients' spiritual lives, accounts of those who claimed to have obtained peace of mind, or who have prepared for the end of their physical existence. McDowall's account is one of the most closely integrated with the Filipino espiritistas' own perspective of their practices in both the physical and spiritual world, with spiritual growth emphasized as the healer's greatest priority for his clients.

McDowall trained while studying under Labo, whereas Martin received his mediumship training from Benjamin Pajarillo. Martin produced an extensive body of work resulting from 10 years of research, which included the perspective of the espiritistas' themselves. Whereas McDowall did not attempt to explain the procedures according to the scientific method or any Western psychological theory, Martin elaborated on the placebo effect/ response. Martin's writings exemplified the changing worldview from the psychical investigations to the perspective of complementary and alternative medicine. Martin emphasizes both self-reports of the espiritistas and the legitimacy of possible placebo effects.

Martin's (1998) book, *The Secret Teachings of the Espiritistas*, provides the most extensive information on the Union of Espiritistas of the Philippines to date. During Martin's time spent in the Philippines, he had early documents of the Union translated into English and has documented a history of the Union of Espiritistas in his book. Martin provides in-depth information regarding the practice of psychic surgery, with less of a parapsychological perspective than previous authors.

> During the mediumship training, the Holy Spirit would initiate the operation of spiritual gifts through the medium. Some would write while in trance; others learned to operate the apparatus in trance; others learned to heal in trance; and still others learned to speak in trance. Such training may take many years, or a few weeks depending upon the existing predisposition of the medium. Yet, with the aid of a qualified instructor, the medium candidate will eventually learn to function in deep trance. Among the Filipinos, this spiritual opening, which allows someone to function in trance, is called *nabuksan* (the opening.) The role of the mediumship trainer is to instruct, guide, and monitor the development of the medium until *nabuksan* takes place. In order to do this, the trainer must be endowed with special gifts of insight and discernment. (Martin, 1998, p. 128)

Martin (1999) posted his article, *Unraveling the Enigma of Psychic Surgery*, on his Web site. His article provides the history of psychic surgery in the Philippines. He also presented the main points of his book, *The Secret Teachings of the Espiritistas* (1998), in the article. He elaborated on several points made in his earlier work. He provided excellent anecdotal material and included explanations not covered in his 1998 book. Following his literature search in Northern Luzon, Martin (1999) provided early documented accounts from the time when the Philippines were in the process of colonization by the Spanish.

> In 1565, a Spanish priest/explorer, Pedro Chirino, described the earliest reference to the therapeutic use of sleight-of-hand in the Philippines. Chirino writes, 'He (the sorcerer) placed one end of the hollow bamboo upon the afflicted part while through the other end he sucked up the air; then, he let fall some pebbles from his mouth, pretending they had been extracted from the afflicted spot.' In 1588, an English explorer, named Cavendish, writes, 'The

priests of these tribes were the sorcerers or medicine men and crude beyond measure was their art in curing, consisting generally of the imaginary extraction of pebbles, leaves, and pieces of cane from the afflicted part.' (p. 4)

Although Martin provided some material on pre-Christian shamanic healing, he referred to the practice of psychic surgery by the Union of Espiritistas of the Philippines, a group of Western influenced spiritualists, as being distinctly different from the traditional Filipino shamanic practices (H. Martin, personal communication, January 18, 2002). Martin provided the most extensive presentation of the belief system of the Filipinos by having old documents written by the founders of The Union of Espiritistas translated into English.

Martin (2000a) elaborated extensively on the system of healing, as perceived by the psychic surgeons themselves, in his self published translation of *A Short Spiritist Doctrine: The History, Beliefs, and Healing Practices of the Spiritist Healers of the Philippine Islands*. The original text had been published in 1909 by J. Obdell Alexis, the founder of the Union of Espiritistas; Martin added a brief introduction to his translation. *The Christian Spiritist Commentaries: Awakening to the Healing Presence of the Spirit of Truth* (2000b) also includes translated writings of Alexis. Both books contain documented accounts of conversations with spirits through mediums, similar to Allen Kardec's (1989) *The Spirit's Book*, which fueled the spiritist movement in Europe and the United States in the late 1800s, and, eventually, in Brazil and the Philippines.

Martin (2002a) has additionally written an article in three parts titled: 'The Origins and Philosophy of Filipino Christian Spiritism, Parts One, Two and Three." These informative articles were written for a new magazine with Jaime Licauco as the senior editor, but they are unpublished at this time (H. Martin, personal communication, January 18, 2002). In these three articles, Martin elaborated on the history of Spiritism and the formation of Christian Spiritism or True Spiritism in the Philippines. Martin concluded these articles with the statement,

"Perhaps the missing context is a paradigm shift into a new spiritual dispensation that has labored long and hard and finally come" (2002a).

Martin reported that most of the written information he gathered while in the Philippines he obtained from the family of Tony Agpaoa. The information was primarily older newspaper articles, but it also included a small booklet written by Agpaoa himself in 1972, *The Gifts of the Spirit* (Martin, 2002b), the only book ever written by a Filipino psychic surgeon. Martin obtained the copyright to publish *The Gifts of the Spirit*, adding an introduction and commentary. The book explains the espiritistas' belief system and their healing practices, which are mostly drawn from the bible. Much of Agpaoa's book is a verbatim compilation of biblical verses, scriptures, and psalms. The book concludes with a section of scriptures translated from the Aramaic Bible, the oldest known manuscript of the bibles, written in the ancient language of the Middle East.

A series of popular books by paranormal investigators and psychical researchers began in the late 1950s and lasted through the 1970s. These authors made many speculations on how psychic surgery worked, but they were all inconclusive. Krippner (1976), a parapsychologist, speculated on several theories, yet, he promoted the idea that the espiritistas generally were healing through therapeutic sleight-of-hand, by stimulating the placebo effect in the patients. The New Age movement in the 1980s offered more inconclusive information, since the practitioners seemed unconcerned with basing their beliefs on any scientific evidence or within any academic discipline. Few anthropologists ever researched psychic surgery, but two authors did contribute a total of three journal articles that provided important information from an anthropological perspective (Lieban, 1981, 1996; Singer, 1990).

Several books were written by practitioners of alternative medicine, who emphasized the perspectives of the espiritistas themselves (Martin, 1998, 1999, 2000a, 2000b, 2002a, 2002b; McDowell, 1998). This view, which did not fully develop until the last decade, is the most congruent with the parameters for complementary and alternative medicine, as presented to the NIHOAM in 1997, the framework for which this author applied the body of knowledge in this study.

The popular trend of complementary and alternative medicine ascended to a new level of legitimacy for Westerners in the 1990s. This new acceptance was exemplified in part by the growing inclusion by the health insurance industry of certain treatments by practitioners of alternative medicine. The budget for the National Institutes of Health's Office of Complementary and Alternative Medicine grew from $2 million in 1992 to $12 million in 1997 (OAM Budget Update, 1997). In October of 1998, the National Institutes of Health Office of Alternative Medicine expanded and became the National Center for Complementary and Alternative Medicine **(NCCAM).**

# III. ARCHIVAL DATA

## Personal Experience

I traveled to the Philippines in January of 2000 and May of 2001. I conducted interviews and acted as a participant-observer with numerous Filipino healers locally referred to as *tambalans*. According to Rebecca Tiston (1983), author of *The Tambalans of Northern Leyte*, the most literal English translation for tambalan is "medicine man" (or "medicine person," as there is a high percentage of females in the profession). On the island of Cebu, I observed approximately 10 local tambalans' activities, conducted interviews with several healers, and participated in treatment. Although their practices are not identical to those of the psychic surgeons of Northern Luzon, many tambalans induce altered states of consciousness and perform as espiritistas.

During my travels in the Philippines in 2000, I asked the healers questions during my interactions with them regarding their callings, initiations, training, and the nature of their work as neighborhood practitioners (see Personal Experience in the Archival Data section), which includes Kleinman's techniques for culturally sensitive interviews). I found the tambalans' stories remarkably similar to the accounts given by the espiritistas from Northern Luzon (see Philippines literature review). I received treatment as a Western participant-observer both from the local tambalans and from a well known psychic surgeon in the Philippines in May of 2001. I had the opportunity to receive treatment from psychic surgeon Emilio Laporga, an espiritista who was originally a member of the Union of Espiritistas of the Philippines in Northern Luzon (the espiritistas who are famous for their practice of psychic surgery). Licauco (1999), Richard Lieban (1981, 1996), McDowall (1998), and others have written about Laporga.

My wife, Dolores Taubold, and other local Filipinos who are related to me by marriage, acted as translators and cultural buffers; they made it possible to interact with the tambalans. These local Cebuanos who were my guides were familiar with the tambalans. Some lived near them and had received treatment from them. One tambalan was related to my wife through marriage. Dolores was familiar with one tambalan who was a close friend of her father. She had previously been treated successfully by him for gallstones. She frequently brought Chinese patients from Cebu City to another neighborhood tambalan who lived behind her family home in the Labogon barrio in Mandaue City. These Cebuanos were also able to verify statements made by the tambalans and to add corroborative and supplemental information regarding their alleged healing practices.

## The Patients

When a person experiences an illness in the Philippines, there are numerous choices of treatment from among the varied healing specialists, both biomedical and alternative healing methods. People form long lines to receive treatment from the tambalans. Healing without pharmaceuticals is the preferred method of treatment of most Filipinos. This choice is made due to the perceived efficacy of their folk-healing systems, as well as the lack of-and high cost of- pharmaceutical medicine. The Philippine Islands abound in folk healers with a wide range of specialties. These services include herbal remedies, massage (and other physical manipulations of the body, such as bone setting), midwifery, prayer or incantations, spiritual interventions, sorcery (malign magic), fortune telling, and more.

Many Filipinos experience their social worlds predominantly in *barrios*. The barrios are political and social units that are spread out over the numerous islands, some metropolitan, but mostly in rural areas.

These neighborhood communities have strong familial ties supported through several generations. The barrios are a continuation of Filipinos' previous tradition of living in kinship groups. Nearly every barrio has a tambalan, although commonly patients will go to tambalans from the neighboring barrios. These neighborhood practitioners are still conducting archaic forms of healing that have been passed from generation to generation.

Life in the rural areas of the Philippines has a timeless quality where beliefs about illness and healing practices, which are centuries old, still remain and constitute the dominant system of healing. In more urban areas, religious, cultural, and healing practices of archaic times often remain intact and coexist with modern methods. The Philippines were a Spanish colony for more than 3 centuries and then were annexed as a territory of the United States as spoils of the Spanish-American War that ended in 1898. The Philippines are modernized and Westernized in the large urban centers. I observed modern Western medicine practiced here, in contrast with alternative medical practices and age-old indigenous practices as well.

One particular event seems to have made a tremendous impact on the healing practices in Cebu since Spanish contact. In 1565, King Philip II of Spain sent Miguel Lopez de Legazpi on an expedition from a Mexican port to the Philippines, where Legazpi settled on the Island of Cebu. The Cebuano chieftain, Tupas, fought him in numerous skirmishes. The day after a particular battle, the Cebuano chieftain burned the Spanish stronghold (which is now Cebu City), and a Spaniard found the image of the infant Jesus, which Magellan had given to a previous chieftain's wife 44 years before. The image was unburned and untarnished. The Filipinos and the Spanish both perceived this as a miracle, and it is reported this occurrence brought about a lasting treaty between them (Agoncillo, 1974).

Legazpi re-named the settlement "City of the Most Holy Name of Jesus." Santo Ninio, the child Christ, became the patron saint of Cebu. Santo Ninio is known for his powerful healing energy. Every year in

January a festival is celebrated in his honor called Sinulog. Sinulog is the celebration of Christianity (Catholicism) coming to the Philippines. The introduction of Christianity in the Philippines has had a major impact on the indigenous healing practices and included the appropriation of the Holy Spirit and the Saints. Many Filipinos believe the Holy Spirit to be a universal healing power. Many of the practitioners refer to this healing power as the Spirit of Santo Ninio, the healing saint of Cebu (Agoncillo, 1974, pp. 39- 40).

During the January celebration of Sinulog, dancers carry images of Santo Ninio. People from all over the Philippines come in dance groups to participate in a parade celebrating their own varied indigenous cultural backgrounds, as well as the healing power of Santo Ninio. The largest church in the city of Cebu is the Church of Santo Ninio. In the churchyard, candles are given to dancers who are standing in lines. They pray and dance while appearing to be in light trance states. The dancers perform this ritual as a method of insuring health or healing for specific individuals who request their service. One can request this service, purchase candles, and inform the dancers of the names of the people in need of prayer. Each candle is blessed with a person's name. The dancer blesses the candles while dancing and returns them to the family, who then burns the candles either at the church or in their home.

## The Healers

Richard Lieban (1967) is an anthropologist, researcher, and author of numerous journal articles and the book, *Cebuano Sorcery: Malign Magic in the Philippines*. His writings were based on two periods of field research in the Philippines. The first, from 1958 to 1959, which took place on Negros Island, was supported by a Fulbright grant. The second period of research, which took place from 1962 to 1963 in Cebu City, was funded by the National Science Foundation. The focus of Lieban's research was health and medicine. Lieban spent a great deal of time in the Philippine Islands, writing extensively on the topics of health care and healing practices there. I made trips to the Island of Cebu on two separate occasions in 2000 and 2001, researching Filipino faith healing. I observed that there has been minimal change in the healing practices since Lieban conducted his research approximately 30 years ago.

The words *tambalan* and *mananambal,* both Visyan words, are interchangeable and have essentially the same meaning. Rebecca Tiston (1983), author of *The Tambalans of Northern Leyte,* refers to the folk healers as tambalans, whereas Lieban (1967) and Martin (1998) refer to the healers as mananambal. The most literal translation for the word *tambalan* is medicine man (or medicine person), whereas *mananambal* is simply translated as doctor. Western trained doctors are not referred to as mananambal. Only the neighborhood practitioners are referred to as mananambal or tambalan. There appear to be no distinct differences in the terminology or practices of these folk healers on the Island of Cebu.

Both Lieban (1967) and Martin (1998) acknowledge that the most popular form of medicine is provided by the tambalans or mananambals, who are considered general practitioners by most Cebuanos. However, some of these general practitioners also engage in the practice of sorcery, acts of inflicting an illness or even death on individuals allegedly guilty of moral injustice. Lieban reports that most of the mananambal he knew were not sorcerers. This is consistent with my experience with the tambalans as well.

Lieban (1967) observed that some mananambal practice sorcery. He reports, "According to sorcerer lore, one becomes a sorcerer by learning methods of malign magic and establishing a relationship with a spirit who supports this magic" (p. 20). When someone has treated another person wrongly, the victim may feel justified in a malevolent act of retribution toward another individual. Bringing about retribution requires hiring a mananambal who doubles as a sorcerer. These pre-Christian methods for retribution utilize the assistance of nature spirits and dark powers, and they originated as indigenous practices that for centuries existed as explanations for illnesses. One female tambalan on

Mactan Island (across the port from Cebu) stated, "There are many sorcerers on Mactan who would like to 'hex' me, but I am protected" (B. Senomio, personal communication, May 15, 2001).

According to Lieban (1967) and my own experience in the Philippines in 2000 and 2001, many of the Filipinos fear sorcery and believe pre-Christian practices utilizing nature spirits are the work of Satan. Lieban articulated the differences among mananambal that seem to be the most meaningful to the Filipinos. He made a clear distinction between mananambal who do practice sorcery and mananambal who do not practice sorcery. Pre-colonial Filipinos commonly practiced sorcery and mediumship while allegedly possessed by spiritual forces. Many Filipinos fear sorcerers. The concern of the local clientele is that they will mistakenly seek treatment from a sorcerer.

Some practitioners claim to heal with the power of God the Father. The incorporation of the Holy Spirit, Santo Nino (God the Son), and God the Father into local mediumship has not completely divorced practitioners from their old beliefs and practices. Their systems of healing most likely have resulted in a compromise. Visiting a tambalan who practiced sorcery was a major concern of the local Cebuanos who escorted me while visiting tambalans on the island of Cebu. However, the fear of sorcerers may well exceed the prevalence of the actual practice.

## The Illnesses

Illness experiences are sometimes perceived as a result of *barang*, a common practice of sorcerers who cast spells resulting in insects entering the victim's body. (I did not hear any firsthand accounts of this particular form of sorcery from my local contacts.) Lieban (1967) explains:

> Barang is the most frequently mentioned form of sorcery in the Cebuano area as a whole. Sometimes the term is employed generically for sorcery; at other times it refers to a specific type of

malign magic in which insects or other animals are sent into the body of a victim by the sorcerer. (p. 50)

Negative energy from a sorcerer can also take the form of objects such as rocks, ferns, rope, shells, and so on placed in the body of the victims of sorcery.

Another well-known condition is referred to as *buyag*. My wife, Dolores Taubold, has often referred to this condition of buyag. A compliment from a *buyagan* (a person or spirit who is capable of emanating buyag, hexes or spells that cause illness) can result in negative effects on one's heath. This type of curse may be placed on a victim by the spoken word. "Buyag is a curse emanating from a compliment rather than an imprecation" (Lieban, 1967, p. 72). Children are particularly subject to the praise of a buyagan, with damaging results.

Buyag is a concern Dolores had frequently expressed regarding our child who was 4 years of age in 2001. Our daughter had taken ill one evening; she had a fever and was crying. Dolores hurried to the neighbor's house and returned with her aunt, the family member with the most folk healing knowledge, to check the child for the spell of a buyagan. Her aunt inspected the child's body from the top of her head to the bottoms of her feet. With her face near the child she made spitting sounds with her mouth. After she made the inspection, she assured my wife there had been no hex placed on our daughter by a buyagan. Our daughter fell asleep and appeared to be symptom-free the next morning. Dolores had attempted to explain the condition of buyagan to me several times. It wasn't until I read Lieban's explanation that I understood the concept.

Practices within the Filipino folk healing systems differ considerably. Folk healers, each with their individual cultural makeup, influence the illness and healing experiences that reflect the worldview of their Filipino patients and their belief systems. Many Filipinos claim to perceive spiritual energies that affect physical reality (Lieban, 1967; Tiston, 1983). The tambalans perceive illnesses in a larger spiritual and metaphysical context than Westerners. Many Filipinos also believe in the existence of another world where God co-exists with nonhuman spirits and the souls of the departed. One must remain in harmony with these entities to sustain a sense of wellness. Disharmony with these beings can bring about distress and discordance that can result in illness.

Tambalans may respond to treat physical complaints rather than spiritual maladies. However, they usually view the etiology within a spiritual and metaphysical perspective. A core belief is that negative energy may manifest in a specific area or organ in the physical body. Sometimes the explanation for the illness is sorcery or hexing.

Conceptions of illness origins are diverse. An illness may have important meaning to the patient and practitioner or it may be the manifestation of a random metaphysical event. The illness may be a result of moral or spiritual failing, a result of a family curse, or the failure to conform to a cultural norm. If the patient is determined to be in need of an intervention, the intervention can take place on either the spiritual/metaphysical or the physical level or both. The whole person will be treated generally, not only an individual part (organ, limb, etc.) of the person. The competent tambalan is able to provide all necessary interventions, herbal cures, massage, the lifting of hexes, spiritual interventions, predicting the future, and so on.

Patients may approach the healer with a previous diagnosis from a Western-trained physician or a family member with some knowledge of folk-healing. It is the tambalan that will ultimately decide the nature of the illness and usually provides immediate treatment for it. The illness may be physical, metaphysical, or spiritual in nature. The illness may be a social or an internal problem caused by a greater corresponding spiritual or metaphysical condition. The illness is generally perceived as a result of both internal and external forces involving the whole person (holistic) rather than merely a specific part of a person.

"According to folk belief, the tambalan has supernatural powers to control the spirits" (Tiston, 1983, p. 3). Illness caused by spiritual forces cannot be cured by modern practitioners but only by the tambalan. My wife (D. Taubold, personal communication, December 1, 2000), an educated Filipina immigrant who worked in California as a certified nursing assistant for 5 years, explained to me, "If a person's illness is due to natural causes, then a doctor can heal the illness; but if a sorcerer caused the illness, it takes a 'faith healer' or sorcerer to remove it."

The allopathic practitioner has advanced modern technologies at her/his fingertips, and with a stroke of the pen can prescribe the most current (and expensive) pharmaceutical medications. These resources are not available to the tambalan. Urban allopathic practitioners have been influenced by Western culture and have largely adopted a Western worldview. A Cebuano's first choice in medical care is generally the tambalan, due to the trust and rapport that comes from their shared worldview. Patients usually come to the tambalan with discomfort or with health concerns. The tambalan diagnoses the problem according to his or her expertise. Patients accept their diagnoses easily, often without question.

The Cebuano tambalans are mainly taught healing by their elders and utilize various folk healing traditions of their local culture. The tambalans may act as espiritistas or mediums, or they may be classified in any of the other categories described in Winkelman's (1992) schema (see Discussion section). Water, oil, and other medications are blessed by the tambalan while channeling the Holy Spirit and these substances are often utilized in treatment within a ritual context. Treatment often consists of herbal medicine supposedly blessed by the Holy Spirit, and may include massage or other minor physical manipulations of the patient's body.

## The Healing Transactions

The roadways in the Philippines made even short journeys to the barrios difficult, as they are in extreme disrepair. After a day of traveling on these roads, I felt aches and pains all over my body. Most people rely on tricycles (small motorcycles with side-carts) or old dilapidated taxi cabs, only some of which have air-conditioning. It is difficult for Westerners to use the small tricycles comfortably, because Westerners tend to be much larger physically than the general Filipino population. I was often required to pay a double fare, because I took up so much room and weighed as much as two local Filipinos.

The neighborhood tambalans were not easily distinguished from the rest of the population, as they, too, lived in the old run down buildings. They dress casually, and there is nothing about their physical appearance that would distinguish them from the other local Filipinos.

Tambalans are known by reputation within the local community and are recognized by their altars, shrines, or chapels. The tambalan's altar or chapel, a sacred space for healing, includes many religious pictures, symbols, and candles that are lit during the healing transactions. Healing chapels in Cebu looked remarkably similar to Alex Orbito's chapel, as viewed in Harvey Martin's video production *Psychic Surgeon of the Philippines, Alex L. Orbito* (Martin, 1985). In Cebu, almost all altars and chapels include images of Santo Ninio and other religious icons similar to those depicted in McDowall's (1998) book *Healing: Doorway to the Spiritual World*. There are frequently sets of three candles representing the Holy Trinity (God the Father, God the Son, and God the Holy Spirit), among the array of other religious artifacts.

While waiting in lines outside the tambalans' healing chapels, patients exchange stories regarding the supposedly effective treatments received by the practitioners. This is how they exchange information about the effectiveness of the tambalans. Word of mouth is very important. People bring water and oil to the shrines to be blessed by the tambalan prior to the healing transactions. Tambalans bless their medicines and will even bless Western pharmaceuticals prior to patients ingesting them. The tambalan often dips his or her fingers in one or more blessed oils and draws a cross on the patient's forehead or back before diagnosing or treating. Tambalans claim that spirit guides assist them in gathering information and diagnosing while they are touching the patients.

Most tambalans utilize the technique of *pulse taking*. "The tambalan takes the pulse of the right hand. The same thing is done with the left. If there is any difference noted, the tambalan interprets it as due to a degree of affliction suffered" (Tiston, 1983, p. 9). A slow or weak pulse indicates low blood pressure and general debility of body and spirit. An intermittent pulse is common among weak and dying patients. A jumpy or spasmodic pulse denotes anxiety, fright, and other emotional disturbances. Rapid or fast pulse indicates severe headache or high blood pressure.

Healing by touch or the laying on of hands is one of the oldest forms of healing in recorded history. The ramifications of the healing power of touch have yet to be defined (Krippner & Remen, 2000). Sometimes the tambalans will touch the center of the chest, lower back, shoulders, and neck to obtain more specific diagnostic information. The tambalan will generally massage the client as needed. Rubbing blessed oil on the body is often practiced. Tambalans generally are very personable and touch their patients frequently. While acting as a channel for the healing power of the Holy Spirit, most practitioners personally manage all aspects of the healing transaction.

Most tambalans use prayer as an integral part of their healing interventions. Amulets made of folded images or other small figures and water and/or coconut oil, which are blessed during the process, are often used. Many tambalans also use herbal remedies. The most common herbals are palm leaves or guava leaves applied to the skin, or *noni* juice to be taken orally. In the Philippines, most people are knowledgeable about herbal remedies, making formal training unnecessary. The blessing of medicines is also common practice for tambalans. Many of the tambalans made similar claims. They have clients who may come all the way from Manila or Luzon, Mindanao, and Leyte. They claim to be able to heal cancer and have had Europeans travel there seeking and receiving cancer treatment.

Catholicism is deeply embedded in the culture and largely influences the dynamics of folk healing practiced on the Island of Cebu. Sin is generally believed to be the cause of illness. Sin is a very general term that can include a vast number of thoughts and behaviors. However, sin can also be conceptualized as thoughts and behaviors that separate the individual from God. It is believed that man's true nature is to be one with, or in communion with, God. This results in the experience of wellness. The role of the patients during the actual healing is to repent for their sins, or to remove sinful thoughts, and to request forgiveness for their behaviors that have separated them from God; then the Holy Spirit can perform a healing process upon patients.

There are usually many deliberate ritual acts performed during the course of treatment. The patient's role is passive, for the most part, during the healing transaction, although the person may be asked to participate in some type of ritual over the course of several days. Patients may drink holy water or rub oil on themselves. They may be required to ingest written prescriptions, either by chewing the paper or by drinking water from containers that contain the prescription. Patients may also be asked to repent for their sins and to go and sin no more. Patients may be asked to perform a follow up ritual at home. Prayer or incantations are generally a part of all rituals.

The tambalan may pray or engage in other ritual acts as a method of healing. They believe the Holy Spirit is responsible for the healing. Patients participate in their own healing process through repentance and improving their relationship with God. Patients are generally present for the healing transactions; however, tambalans do perform distance healing through prayer, perhaps while engaging in one of the above-mentioned ritual practices. In most cases, patients are informed of how and when the distance healing will be performed. The failure to heal is often perceived as God's will. This is acceptable when it is believed that God possesses infinite wisdom, and human beings are lacking wisdom in relation to the spirit world and the afterlife.

The tambalans on the island of Cebu generally restrict their healing transactions to Tuesdays, Fridays, and sometimes Sundays, which are considered to be Holy Days. Practitioners who are unable to provide service to all their patients in that time frame may make themselves available to provide services on other days during the week. Tambalans usually refrain from providing services during times of fiesta, election weeks, and other occasions when a shift in spiritual energies may effect their healing transactions. The healing sessions of many of the patients take place within only a few minutes at the tambalan's altar. The tambalan usually keeps a rigorous schedule, as people wait in line for their treatments. It can be observed that healers become tired and even physically exhausted after more than half a day of performing healing transactions one right after another.

The services performed by the tambalans are not just concerned with symptom alleviation. The goals of their healing processes are to bring the patient into a state of holistic balance and facilitate involvement in spiritual development. They generally treat the whole person, although specific areas of physical concern are commonly addressed. The tambalan may detect concerns different from the patients' perceptions of the illness or their reported symptoms. Restoration of physical, emotional, and spiritual health is the shared goal of patient and practitioner working together with the intervening power of the Holy Spirit. Regarding the healing relationship, Tiston (1983) refers to aspects of the Torrey Model, (as described in the Literature review: System of Healing Models):

> The methods used by psychic healers have the same mechanism with that of the psychologists and psychiatrists in healing psychotic patients. Usually the tambalan can cure more than just physical ailments. He is able to locate lost objects or stolen property, divine future events, assure personal success in personal matters as well as success in business, cure insanity and counteract the affects of witchcraft. (pp. 6-12)

Tambalans are not well-compensated monetarily on the island of Cebu. Practitioners within this indigenous healing system have accepted an obligation to heal others, generally, out of compassion, and they recognize only minimal compensation for their efforts. The compassion of the healers is strongly supported by Christian belief.

Ministering to others is a highly valued Christian ideal in Filipino culture. Although many Filipinos do not value this particular system of healing, the tambalans are highly esteemed by the patients who do utilize their services. The tambalans are often referred to as *quack doctors* by the more Westernized Filipinos, who prefer to receive services from Western-trained medical professionals.

Most healers accept a donation for their service, in whatever amounts patients feel they can afford to pay. Most practitioners do not openly request payment. They have a cup or bowl on the altar where payments can be deposited after a healing transaction. I experienced one tambalan refusing to accept a donation; however, his wife had earlier solicited donations as a contribution for the upcoming fiesta. One tambalan specified the amount of a donation after performing what he referred to as a psychic surgery. He had not performed a psychic surgery as such, but had only administered a superficial skin treatment.

This same tambalan, who referred to himself as a psychic surgeon, originally came from the island of Mindinao. He apparently performed minor surgeries and other techniques similar to that of the Luzon healers, such as Emilio Laporga. According to one Filipina patient's personal testimony, the surgeon had dissolved lumps on her breasts (perhaps through magnetic healing). My wife, Dolores, her brother (who had been circumcised at 8 years of age without anesthetic), and I were asked to leave towards the end of the morning healing session as the tambalan was to perform a circumcision on a young boy. This particular tambalan was not comfortable being observed by a Westerner, even when accompanied by the local Filipinos.

## Emilio Laporga

I found Emilio Laporga's address while in Cebu City, located his clinic, and had the opportunity to receive treatment from him in May of 2001. Laporga has practiced for nearly 30 years at his clinic, adjacent to his large modern home at Tiza, Labangon, Cebu City, Philippines.

According to Licauco (1999), who had also been treated at the clinic, the house had been donated to Laporga by a grateful patient who he had cured in 1973. Laporga relocated to his modern home in Cebu from the Pangasinan region in Northern Luzon, where the majority of the psychic surgeons practiced a similar form of Kardec-influenced spiritism, mediumship, and psychic surgery.

According to the Kardec-influenced espiritistas, not all diseases or discomforts require psychic surgery. There are times when the espiritistas perform magnetic healing on a patient or merely massage the afflicted part with blessed oil, channeling the healing power of the Holy Spirit. If a patient requires surgery, it is reported that the fingers and/or the hands of the espiritista apparently enter the body wall with a kneading motion, which often creates a popping sound as the flesh is penetrated. In some reports it appears that diseased tissue materializes on the surface of the body without any body wall penetration. Reports of other psychic surgeons, such as Blanche and Laporaga, allege that they perform distance cutting with a stroke of the finger from several feet away. In my experience, Laporga utilized a surgical instrument to cut the skin open in order to extract tissue.

It is reported by several sources (Licauco, 1999; McDowall, 1998) that some of the prominent Filipino espiritistas (Terte and Labo) had at first used knives to perform surgeries similar to Arigo's technique in Brazil. The early practitioners found they were exempt from prosecution by the medical and legal authorities in the Philippines, as long as they did not use instruments to perform their surgeries and instead use their bare hands. Laporga apparently began using surgical instruments later in his life, between the years of 1990 and 2001.

Laporga had made many cultural adaptations over the years. His operating room included an image of the local healing saint, Santo Ninio, reflecting his embrace of Cebuano's traditional Christian healing tradition. Earlier in his career, he claimed to heal with the help of his spirit guide, "a woman dressed in white," the spirit of Mary Magdalene. He reported to me his healing power was that of the Holy Spirit, which is the most common explanation for healing powers in Cebu City. I visited Laporga at his clinic twice in May of 2001 as a patient. In his large waiting room, which needed fresh paint, was a framed series of photographs showing the process of the removal of a large cyst that covered the entire upper back and shoulders of a Filipino. A caption read "Painless Surgery Without Anesthetics or Bleeding."

A Filipina who acted as an assistant to Laporga met us at the door. She asked a few questions prior to escorting patients into the three-bed operating room. I initially asked her if I could observe Laporga's practice, take photographs and, perhaps, a video. She went back into the room for a moment to consult with him and then returned, escorting us into the operating room. Laporga suggested that if I wished to observe psychic surgery that, perhaps, I should observe by receiving treatment myself. I admitted to him that I had a lot of health problems. He said, "I know." He pointed to the many lipomas (epidermal fatty cysts) on my forearms and suggested that I let him remove one. I also told him later I had diabetes, for which he provided treatment by rubbing oils on my abdomen.

Although a foreigner to Philippine culture, I had a deep interest in obtaining some hard data on the practice of psychic surgery. I had previously had two lipomas removed by conventional biomedical means with the use of anesthetics in Aiea, Hawaii. I felt that having Laporga remove one of my lipomas would make good primary research. Since I had a similar procedure before, I could make a comparison between the two treatments, conventional biomedical surgery and psychic surgery in the Philippines.

In spite of the fact there were only a few patients in the clinic on that day, Laporga did not want to perform the treatment at that time. Laporga said he had only recently returned from a training seminar in Mexico, and his patients did not know yet that he had returned. He asked me to return in 2 days for the treatment. I was unaware of the significance of his timing of appointments 2 days prior to and 2 days following treatment. I later determined this to be a pattern to which he wished to adhere. I had a previous engagement at that time, so we settled on one week from that day. We had to wait for election week to pass, because of the belief that these types of sociopolitical events can manifest energy that can affect healers' abilities and/or their treatment outcomes. Following the treatment, he asked me to return in 2 days for a follow-up visit.

Licauco (1999) reports Laporga's techniques are nearly identical to Blanche's, with whom Laporga had apprenticed during the 1960s. Similar to Blanche, Laporga incorporated other indigenous healing techniques in his practice, such as the ancient art of cupping (see Other Reported Phenomena in the 1970s section). While at Laporga's clinic, I observed one Caucasian male receiving cupping treatments while I was on the next bed. Laporga explained that this patient came in regularly for this treatment for his back pain. The other patient in the operation room was a Filipina, apparently being treated for lumps on her breasts. He worked by reaching up under her t-shirt, apparently due to the lack of privacy. Therefore, I was unable to view this particular treatment procedure.

Laporga was quiet while providing the treatments. I had to ask questions to get him to speak at all. He rubbed oils on my abdomen for the treatment of diabetes. During my stay, and for 2 weeks after, my blood sugar levels did decrease, but one could attribute that change to the change in diet and/or climate that I experienced during my stay in the Philippines. Laporga did not perform distance cutting on me as documented in previous reports of his practice, but utilized a razor knife, scissors, cotton balls, alcohol, a bowl, and small glass cups for the cupping procedure while performing treatment on me and the other patients I observed.

Laporga removed a benign lipoma from my left forearm. As mentioned previously, I had had lipomas on my forearms removed at a Hospital in Aiea, Hawaii. Both experiences were somewhat painful. Laporga's treatment did include some pain at the first point of incision, as he cut through the skin above the lipoma with a razor-knife. However,

Laporga's operation, in which he claimed to utilize the Holy Spirit as anesthetic, was significantly less painful than the conventional allopathic treatment, which included a local anesthetic. Laporga's operation did not require cauterization, as did the conventional treatment, which was extremely painful, and I did not experience any swelling or discoloration afterward. During the middle of the operation, Laporga, a showman, raised up my arm so I could view the lipoma half-way removed, while my wife recorded the entire operation on video.

Upon my return to the clinic 2 days later, Laporga released me from his care. As we stood together to speak afterward, Laporga stated, "I could make your wife more beautiful by removing the mole on her face." He again requested that we return in 2 days. We informed him that we were leaving the Philippines very soon and could not meet this time schedule. He agreed to perform the procedure and told Dolores to lay down on one of the operating tables. Laporga performed cosmetic surgery on Dolores's face, removing several moles, one on her nose very near her eye, and they have never returned. Because Dolores had been treated successfully by the local Filipino healers on numerous occasions, she was not particularly nervous about the operation.

Laporga used surgical scissors and his razor-knife to make the incisions on the moles; he called upon the power of the Holy Spirit to act as an anesthetic. I noted that while Laporga performed the surgery on Dolores' face, although he frequently lifted his left hand, whenever he cut with his right hand, his left hand made contact with her body. Similarly, while performing surgery on my left forearm, his left hand was in contact the entire time he operated. The espiritistas report the left hand is always held against the body to continue the flow of magnetic energy. The right hand is used to remove blockages, diseased tissue, or foreign matter. When the left hand is removed, the opening in the body will close.

The procedures Laporga performed on Dolores and me were successful, leaving only tiny scars. The lipoma and the moles have not yet returned. Since that time, I have recommended that fellow Westerners go to the Philippines for treatment for physical ailments, because there is little pain or bleeding. Laporga claimed the successes of his treatments were due to his channeling of the Holy Spirit. Although it is difficult for an observer to determine if or when the espiritistas are entering trance states, the healers conceptualize themselves as channels for the Holy Spirit to perform operations, a process of the Holy Spirit working through the healer. The Holy Spirit works as an "anesthetic," prevents infection, and minimizes bleeding, while guiding the mind and hands of the surgeon during the course of the operation.

Much of the written information I reviewed is consistent with my own experience. According to his assistant, Laporga prepares himself prior to seeing patients by going into trance. While the Holy Spirit is working through him, the surgeon makes a diagnosis (Laporga reported that he knew I had many health problems) and appears to enter the body of the patient with bare hands, or, with minimal use of surgical instruments. Laporga used some small surgical instruments. The surgeon apparently removes tissues or diseased organs from the body and then seems to "close the patient up again" without leaving a scar, or, with only minimal scarring. This was consistent with my experience. Psychic surgery is performed while the patient is fully conscious, and spectators often observe the process. The healing takes place on the operating table and is performed very quickly. This was all consistent with my experience, while acting as a participant-observer with Laporga.

An espiritista's powers will often decrease with age or may be affected by other variables, such as public holidays, election week, and so on. Advanced age might account for Laporga's practice of using the surgical instruments. He had aged 30 years since Lieban's and many others' written accounts reported his utilization of distance cutting and other more dynamic healing methods. Although, in 1990, two public officials reported that Laporga's techniques "involved psychokinetic phenomena" (McDowall, 1998, p. 186). In May of 2001, Laporga still exhibited the ability to perform psychic surgery, supposedly by channeling the Holy Spirit for anesthetic and antibiotic effects, as well as for reducing bleeding. He, himself, refers to psychic surgery as a surgical procedure that is "painless and without bleeding."

There are two points that are important to mention from my own personal experience observing the tambalans on the island of Cebu. It was my observation that the expression of an underlying belief system and general practices of the espiritistas in Cebu (tambalans or mananambals) were remarkably similar to the reports of the espiritistas' in Northern Luzon. The only difference between the two groups of practitioners appears to be the phenomenal display of psychic surgery by the Kardec-influenced group of espiritistas.

It is often difficult to determine if, and when, a healer is entering a trance state or alternate state of consciousness (ASC). Since language and conceptual barriers exist, "this determination often requires consistent observations of an individual healer" (R. Heinze, personal communication, September 2, 2000).

I was unable to verify the use of ASC by the tambalans I observed. However, behaviors such as speaking in altered tones of voice, altered facial expressions, and their ritual acts indicated a definite cultural heritage of the use of ASC by the healing practitioners in Cebu.

# IV. METHODOLOGY

## Overview

A number of considerations and constraints influence how a researcher selects an appropriate strategy. The research of alternative medicine, in general, is difficult (at best), as many cultural and linguistic considerations come to bear, with which even the best of researchers must struggle. The present study of psychic surgery represents an endeavor to describe the most radical of almost all alternative methods of medical practice. Standard research methods may not apply; techniques used by psychical researchers are inconclusive; and qualitative measures serve only to a certain extent, as this system of healing is based on faith and, possibly, on paranormal phenomena.

In *Clinical Research in Complementary Therapies: Principles, Problems and Solutions,* Lewith, Jonas, and Walach (2002) contend that:

> Research on alternative medical practices requires the same rigorous methods developed for conventional medicine. These methods include laboratory techniques, observational methods, randomized controlled trials, meta-analysis, qualitative research methods, health-services research and health technology assessment. (p. 8)

Targ (2002) begins to describe her proposed methodology for research on a paranormal healing technique by defining the intervention. Targ contends that one must define specifically what the healing intervention is before further research can occur.

This is a fundamental concern regarding the research of psychic surgery. The espiritistas make claims that are not easily verified by observers. The espiritistas' claims are also not easily verified with the use of standard scientific testing. The practice of psychic surgery has baffled most interested people worldwide for the last half century. The researcher must remain constantly vigilant for bias from personal, cultural, and disciplinary perspectives.

Archival research is the chosen methodology in this study, drawing on a large body of archival information that includes personal accounts by the Filipino espiritistas, observations of Filipinos as patients, Westerners as patients and observers, and the previous personal experiences of this author as well. The object of compiling archival data is to discover and describe (frequently referred to as psychic surgeons). The structured analysis of the components of alternative healing systems will be extremely beneficial to this study of psychic surgery and other indigenous healing systems.

The parameters for complementary and alternative medicine (O'Connor et al., 1997) were employed to produce a detailed description of the essential elements of healing and to obtain a better understanding of the practices of the Filipino espiritistas' system of healing. A variety of systems of healing models are reviewed to provide a context for indigenous healing systems. The research model chosen for this study was generated by the United States National Institutes of Health Office of Alternative Medicine. The systems of healing model used in this study is The Parameters for Complementary and Alternative Medicine (see Appendix A).

> In April 1995, the U. S. Office of Alternative Medicine (OAM) of the National Institutes of Health held a conference on research methodology to evaluate research needs in the large, diverse, and dynamic field of complementary and alternative medicine (CAM). Several working groups were empanelled by the OAM to produce consensus statements on a variety of topics essential to CAM research. The panel on definition and description accepted a dual charge: to establish a definition of the field for CAM purposes of identification and research; and to identify factors critical to thorough and unbiased description of CAM systems and practices

that would be applicable to both quantitative and qualitative research. (O'Connor et al., 1997, p. 49)

Other systems of healing models will be employed for their utility consistent with the findings of this study.

## The Archival Method

The Philippines is a country widely known for its faith healing practices. Yet, their techniques of healing are rarely, if ever, recorded, but are instead passed along as oral tradition, making local archival research extremely difficult. There has also been a lack of serious research performed regarding the indigenous healing practices common to this part of the world. The people of the Philippines have a very long indigenous cultural heritage, yet, at the same time, they have been enormously influenced by colonization by the Spanish and their strict Catholicism and by the influx of modern Western paradigms and technologies.

This author attempted to find literature in local and university libraries on the indigenous folk healing systems while in the Philippines, as well as by searching databases. Language and cultural barriers complicated this process. An extensive literature search was conducted in libraries in both the United States and in Cebu City in the Philippines, which included both primary and secondary resources. Local contacts were obtained with access to the large university libraries in Cebu City. It was determined that written information on indigenous healing practices was nearly nonexistent on the island of Cebu. There is a minimal amount of information published by Filipinos themselves on this subject. Westerners who spent time in the Philippines wrote most of the literature only in the last half century, and nearly all of the available information was published in the United States. Several books from Italy and Australia on the topic of Philippine psychic surgery were also obtained.

To produce a description of the healing system, reports of others were used, as well as my personal observations while acting as a participant-observer in the Philippines, previous to this study. The data were then applied to the CAM parameters. In this study, publications written by persons from a wide range of backgrounds, experience, and theoretical perspectives were utilized. Writings by a parapsychologist, numerous reporters, psychologists, anthropologists, laypersons, and practitioners of both alternative and allopathic medicine were included. These authors' accounts collectively generated a pool of information that resulted in the formation of a more comprehensive description than had previous attempts. The application of the CAM parameters to the review of the literature provided a framework with which to separate out individual bias in the observations and theories of these cross-disciplinary authors, many of whom observed the phenomena of purported psychic surgery.

## Advantages

The archival method is both the science and art of locating, studying, and interpreting primary documents. In this study, the archival data were used to construct corroborating information to assist in the understanding of phenomena. There were definite advantages to the use of archival data in this study. La France (1981) noted "the advantage of using collected data to assess the effects of the natural treatments is economical in the data collection stage" (p. 266). In this study, each author who contributed to the archival data spent individually anywhere from 2 weeks to 8 years in the Philippines. All of this combined time spent is more than any one individual could, perhaps, spend in an entire career of field investigations. The archival data also include very detailed information provided by a local Filipino, Licauco (1977, 1999), who has spent a large portion of his career writing about so-called paranormal healing in the Philippines.

The diverse backgrounds and theoretical approaches of these various investigators' observations have collectively produced a varied and, therefore, presumably unbiased body of information that was then applied to the CAM parameters to produce a description. Most importantly, the healers provided the most vital information regarding their perspectives of their own practices. It is extremely time-consuming to establish rapport and to develop an understanding of concepts cross-culturally. Therefore, the use of archival data was "advantageous and economical" in this study for the reasons noted by La France (1981, p. 266).

Archival sources were well suited to the study of phenomena not amenable to investigation through other means. For example, an advantage of utilizing archival data was that it did not require the cumbersome collection of information directly from individuals. Language differences requiring translation were a most difficult barrier to overcome while performing research in the Philippines. Even with the use of adequate translators, fundamental differences in worldview presented challenges to the researcher, who must also interpret conceptual information regarding the indigenous worldview, including cultural beliefs regarding illness and healing. Therefore, the use of archival data, which included some firsthand experience, was preferred to other methods for a study of this nature. For example, my wife had attempted to explain the concept of buyag, a type of curse that was supposedly placed on our daughter. It was not until I read Lieban's (1967) explanation of the phenomena (see Archival Data section) that I understood the concept.

Language is a major concern addressed by the National Institutes of Health's panel in developing the descriptive parameters for complementary and alternative medicine (CAM). According to O'Connor et al. (1997), clarity and care in articulation of word choice are essential to efforts descriptive of CAM healing systems.

> The language of definition and description must, for professional purposes, be non-evaluative, avoiding implications of favorability.

> Explicitly or implicitly evaluative linguistic choices have both obvious and subtle effects on distribution of research interest and funding, conduct and contours of research studies, legislation and regulatory activity, patterns of practice and usage, policy decisions, and other sequelae of practical consequence. It is challenging to forge appropriate language for definition and description in a field as contested and politically charged, and value-laden as CAM, because these very linguistic acts "presuppose a particular point of view, and often carry a moral tone," and may suggest by their selection of words whether the subject is to be regarded favorably or unfavorably. (p. 50)

Language is particularly challenging when the literature requires translation. In regard to psychic surgery, Martin (1998) explains, "These were complex issues that I could not discuss with the Filipinos because of my limited command of their language" (p. 160). Additionally, cross-cultural understanding of illness and healing concepts reflects an indigenous worldview differing from other frames of reference and is often difficult to grasp. Furthermore, many Filipinos acknowledge Christian spiritism, congruent in some ways with Western Christianity. However, they also have prevalent beliefs in witchcraft, which are not generally taken seriously by Westerners. Neither do many Western-influenced Filipinos nor Westerners view the practice of psychic surgery seriously, so the availability of quality local literature is scarce.

## Disadvantages

As a scientific method, the archival method is based on factual evidence. However, in this study the data were derived from popular books, as well as scholarly journals, private holdings, and public information. The archival method generally consists in discovery, identification, verification, and acquisition of documents, and, in this study, these materials were combined with personal experience. My personal observations are presented as archival data since they were collected prior to this study of the phenomena.

Observations of psychic surgery are influenced by each individual's own belief system and worldview. Certainly, the phenomenon itself is difficult to observe fairly, given that psychic surgery often transcends normal expectations, and, perhaps, represents very talented trickery, leaving the observer uncertain of what was actually taking place. The problem of bias is inherent due to the consistent use of a specific paradigm by which to examine the phenomena. Any given individual brings to the observation his or her varied background, beliefs, and experiences that yield vastly different reports of similar phenomena.

It is important to mention that the content of the archival data compiled for this study was essentially participant observations, with some interviewing by Westerners of the members of the Union of Espiritistas of the Philippines. The observations of individuals' view of psychic surgery are influenced by their own belief system and worldview. It is important to determine authors' biases when reading the popular literature generated by psychic surgery. Individual views of psychic surgery will be influenced by the respective belief system.

Wood (1977) proposed that the function of the observer is to record the behavior of individuals or events that actually occurred. Wood argues, "You may see a rabbit eating dandelions and record that the hungry rabbit ate dandelions. However, it is not clear that the animal was hungry; perhaps it was eating because of boredom, anxiety, or an unresolved oral fixation" (p. 30). C. Van Woodward (1955) elaborated on this issue of reliability in archival research in the essay titled "On Believing What One Reads." He addressed the complexity of this issue stating, "Evidence, therefore, consists not only of 'hard facts' but also of beliefs, for myths widely enough entertained have ways of becoming true" (p. 25). Beliefs or assumptions are frequently specific to various disciplines and are often determined by culture.

Issues of private life and public status become major concerns when the authors stand to gain financially or prestigiously from their accounts of a phenomenon. Woodward (1955) noted, "In truth, not every man can be his own historian, for the gap between decisions made within one's private life and those decisions made in one's public capacity is often dangerously narrow" (p. 29). One must allow for the personal interests of authors while examining the historical data relating to the Filipino espiritistas.

## The Inclusion of Personal Experience in the Archival Data

To conclude this Methodology section, it is important to mention that this author traveled to the Philippines in the years 2000 and 2001 and had opportunities to meet with, speak with, and receive treatment from Filipino espiritistas (several tambalans and one psychic surgeon) on the island of Cebu. My personal account, along with the many other first-person accounts that date back to the late 1950s, have contributed to the body of archival data. I also spoke with many other Filipinos and Westerners who had been treated by the espiritistas. My opportunity for personal participation included observations of the procedures performed on others, experiencing certain procedures on myself, and the opportunity to speak with both local practitioners and patients. These observations enriched this study with important archival data from primary sources. The CAM parameters specify that information included in a description be consistent with the practitioners' views and how they, in this case the espiritistas, perceive their system of healing. The utilization of this framework provided a control for personal, professional, and discipline bias.

I utilized Kleinman's (1980, 1988b) outline for culturally sensitive interviews. He suggests a semistructured, nondirective, person centered approach to assess individual and cultural differences. Klienman contends that universally similar emotions in response to events may present in all societies, but because of the particularities of culture, situation, and person, they will be distinctive to the individual. He promotes a four-stage process for interviewing, which includes empathic listening, translation, interpretation, and negotiation.

He recommends open-ended questions rather than short, closed-ended questions. However, if I asked direct questions such as, "When did you first become a healer?" the question would generally illicit much information regarding callings, initiation, and training from individual practitioners. The close observations of cultural myths translate local customs into terms that enable comparisons. Major economic, psychological, social systems of kinship, and spiritual/religious themes and concepts place in context the individual's changing innerworld. "This process facilitates a more full and accurate disclosure of the patient's model" (Kleinman, 1980, p. 106).

# V. LITERATURE REVIEW: THE SYSTEMS OF HEALING MODELS

## Early Research

The study of spiritism and other types of "psychic phenomena" are not new to the discipline of psychology. For more than a century, several psychologists and parapsychologists have conducted research with spiritualists, mediums, and other psychic claimants. During the 1850s and 1860s, the spiritualist or spiritist movement in Europe grew to enormous proportions. Serious scientific investigation of psychic phenomena has been ongoing since at least 1882, with the founding of the Society for Psychical Research in England (Hansen, 2001; Hess, 1993). Initially, the boundaries between spiritualism and psychical research were not clearly defined. 'The original Society of Psychical Research in Britain included Spiritualists as well as scholars and scientists among its ranks" (Hess, p. 22).

The best known American supporter of psychical research was psychologist and philosopher William James, a graduate of Trinity College (renamed Duke University). This American institution owes much of its early existence to the support of James, who died in 1910. A sharp division between spiritualists and psychical researchers occurred in 1923, when proponents of spiritualism gained control of the American Society for Psychical Research, a spin-off of the British organization (Hess, 1993, p. 8).

Spiritualists have frequently used the term "psychological" to describe their work, rather than "psychic," a term generally applied to more nebulous, unscientific, and marginalized notions. The terms "psychical research" and "psychology" were more or less interchangeable in the late 1800s. At the turn of the century, the relationship of psychical research to psychology-not to mention the meaning of the very terms-was still poorly defined. William James, who maintained a lifelong interest in psychical research, wielded a great influence on American psychology. A major paradigm shift took place with the death of the older generation of psychologists, the advent of behaviorism, and the development of psychotherapeutic procedures such as free association (Hess, 1993, pp. 28-29). However, some psychologists continued to promote the study of mediumship in mainstream psychological communities.

Shortly after this paradigm shift in the discipline of psychology, a division between the spiritualists and psychical researchers happened, as parapsychologists began to utilize increasingly sophisticated technologies in the early 20th century. In 1929, Hans Berger discovered the possibility of measuring the brain's electrical currents through electroencephalography (EEG). The question was proposed, "If electrical currents of a vibratory nature can reach the surface of the skull, then it makes sense that electromagnetic waves and fields in the air around the human head can reach the brains of others" (Stelter, 1976, p. 21). New technologies were applied to the study of the paranormal, supplementing or replacing the case study and observational methods of previous psychical research methodologies.

It was not until the work of J.B. Rhine, at Duke University, in the early 1930s, that the systematic laboratory approach to anomalous phenomena was institutionalized. Rhine's work, and that of his followers, replaced the uncertainties of the case history and observational methods and focused on the laboratory approach with its new technologies. Rhine remained the leader in his field from the 1930s to the 1960s (Hansen, 2001, p. 312). Some of the technologies he experimented with were utilized by other investigators. Some of their accounts are included in the Western literature review section of this study and contribute to the body of information. However, many researchers since Rhine have shifted their focus to a more qualitative system of healing perspective, which is, in some ways, more similar to the early psychological perspective.

## The Systems of Healing Approach

Due to the complexity of human beings' illnesses and healing experiences, several researchers have attempted to determine universal components of these experiences. Many contemporary researchers and theorists have tried to define illnesses and healing experiences, and they have created classifications as to cause and cure, in order to provide descriptions of particular systems of healing. Proponents of the systems of healing perspective believe that not only physical health, but also human consciousness and social and environmental experiences play prominent roles in affecting human illness and healing experiences.

It is necessary to include the use of a systems of healing approach to broaden the research inquiry into spiritism and the phenomena of psychic surgery. The systems of healing approach can be utilized to assist in understanding the effectiveness of indigenous healing systems by answering fundamental questions such as: (a) What cluster of symptoms is considered an illness? (b) What mode of treatment is deemed appropriate? (c) What exactly constitutes healing, the absence of symptoms or progress towards a goal?

Proponents of the systems of healing approach contend that human consciousness, belief systems, and social worlds affect both the experience of illness and the healing process. Many researchers and theorists emphasize social and behavioral components that reflect a wide variety of effective healing systems in which human consciousness plays an essential role (Frank & Frank, 1991; Kleinman, 1980; Krippner & Remen, 2000; O'Connor et al., 1997; Siegler & Osmond, 1974; Torrey, 1972).

The complementary and alternative medicine (CAM) parameters, as presented by O'Connor et al. (1997), utilized in this research are an example in the West of a currently accepted systems of healing model. The parameters focus on CAM systems, rather than biomedicine, psychiatry, or psychotherapy. The parameters allow for the inclusion of socio-cultural factors. The CAM parameters incorporate the same essential elements of illness and healing as the other systems of healing models. An effort to define essential healing principles has a long history among doctors, psychologists, psychotherapists, and professionals in other disciplines as well. The systems of healing approach assists in the evaluation of alternative healing systems.

## Kleinman: Patients and Healers in the Context of Culture

Arthur Kleinman, M.D., Ph.D., a psychiatrist who is also trained in anthropology, provides an excellent framework for identifying specific clinical concepts cross-culturally in *Patients and Healers in the Context of Culture: An Exploration of the Borderland Between Anthropology, Medicine, and Psychiatry* (1980). He emphasizes sensitivity to cultural context, explanatory models of illness and healing, and the clinical realities in which illness experiences occur. Kleinman suggests that illness experiences are affected largely by culture and social interaction. Kleinman's fieldwork in Taiwan from 1968 to 1969 both inspired and provided the opportunity for the development of his theoretical framework in this area of medical and psychiatric anthropology. He continues to research and lecture on healing systems today. Kleinman's perspective is relevant for two important reasons. He focuses on indigenous healing systems and cultural influence, and he explores cultural diversity which blends Eastern, Western, and indigenous healing systems.

Kleinman (1980) states, "Regardless of which society we choose to examine, we would always find people we could identify (and more importantly, whom the local population would identify) as healers and patients" (p.8). Two significant concepts of Kleinman's model are the *clinical reality* and the *illness experience*. The clinical reality is the situation in which symptoms of illnesses may be identified as metaphors and where the treatment for the illness experience takes place. According to Kleinman, health care systems are socially and culturally constructed. Health care systems exist as forms of a social reality, agreed upon as acceptable means of treating illness and disease.

Social reality is a construct that constitutes meanings, institutions, and relationships sanctioned by a given society. "Certain meanings, social structural configurations, and behaviors are sanctioned or legitimated, while others are not" (Kleinman, 1980, p. 36).

> Anthropologist Jilek (1982) also supports this contention:
> Every individual is prepared during the course of his life by a set of expectancies regarding illness and treatment which are a part of his culture. These are inculcated long before his own condition as a patient comes about. They are heightened, however, as he approaches being a patient and increase the suggestive power of many of the experiences he undergoes. (p. 46)

This social and cultural world that Kleinman describes as the social reality links the social/cultural experience and the psychological and biological realities that influence illness and health care. For the specific purposes of examining and understanding illness and healing, Kleinman (1980) developed the concept of "clinical reality" (p. 41).

> In many cultures shamans, herbalists, faith healers, as well as psychotherapists must interpret somatic complaints as bodily icons of troubles in various domains of a person's life (home, work place, school, street, interstices of the self). Healers and patients create a local cultural-ethos of expectations about clinical etiquette, action, and outcome that is referred to as the "clinical reality" of each cultural group (Kleinman, 1980, p. 119).

According to Kleinman (1980), disease and illness are explanatory concepts, not entities. Kleinman goes on to establish an *illness model*. "Disease refers to a malfunctioning of biological and/or psychological processes while the term illness refers to the psychological experience and meaning of a perceived disease "(p. 119). Kleinman contends that if we examine symptomology, it is possible to see just how complex the interrelationship is between disease and illness, as well as health and healing, which are, in turn, individually and collectively influenced by culture. The first manner in which an illness manifests meaning is through a symptom. A symptom is an indicator of illness. Illness usually begins with the sick person's attention to and perception of the early manifestations of disease. A particular event can be experienced as a symptom because the cultural meaning defines it as an indicator of illness (p. 197).

Illness may also begin with a person being labeled ill by others, even though he or she has no subjective complaints. The cultural construction of illness experiences is frequently a personally and socially adaptive response. Illness contains responses to distress and disease, which attempt to provide meaningful explanation and control over the experienced symptoms. In some cultures, the illness is believed to be constituted by both the affected person and his or her family; both are labeled ill. Personal and family beliefs and experiences, and through them culture and social systems, are powerful influences on these processes (Kleinman, 1980, pp. 73- 75).

Richard Castillo (1997), elaborates on Kleinman's explanatory models for illness and healing. Castillo contends that patients and practitioners hold explanatory models in all health care systems.

> Explanatory model refers to the way a set of cultural schemas explains the cause of illness-why the onset occurred when it did, the effects of the illness, what course the illness will take, and what treatments are appropriate. These meanings dramatically affect the lived experiences of people with illnesses, in many ways structuring the subjective illness experience. (p. 35)

Explanatory models offer a narrative for sickness, as well as for guiding treatment choices from among available therapies and therapists. These models also cast personal and social meaning on the experience of sickness. "Structurally, we can distinguish five major categories that explanatory models seek to explain for illness episodes. These are: (1) etiology; (2) time and mode of onset of symptoms; (3) pathophysiology; (4) course of sickness; and (5) treatment" (Kleinman, 1980, p. 105).

Kleinman began his research while performing an internship at a hospital in Taiwan in 1968, where many cultural variables are similar to those in the Philippines. He is currently a professor at Harvard University. He was most likely influenced by both Jerome Frank and E. F. Torrey. In his writings, Kleinman frequently reveals the influence of humanistic psychology. He developed a meaning centered model to assist in establishing an explanatory model of patients' illness experiences. Kleinman frequently mentions a phenomenological perspective. He does not elaborate on a particular phenomenological perspective, only that a phenomenological strategy may be utilized generally while eliciting illness meanings from patients. Kleinman is one of the most influential scholars in the disciplines of social medicine and medical anthropology. He refers to himself as writing across other disciplines and titled his most recent book *Writing at the Margin: Discourse Between Anthropology and Medicine* (1995).

## Frank and Frank: Persuasion and Healing

Jerome Frank, M.D., Ph. D., first published *Persuasion and Healing: A Comparative Study of Psychotherapy* in 1963. His daughter, Julia Frank, M.D., was added as a co-author for the third edition of the book in 1991. The Franks have devoted themselves to observing and understanding psychotherapy. They focused on finding the common denominators that exist in the process of psychotherapy, and the commonalities that can also be found in both indigenous and alternative healing systems.

Frank and Frank trace healing traditions back to a time when illness was regarded as primarily supernatural or magical and when treatment consisted of rituals that reversed the cause of the illness, similar to traditions that are still prevalent in the Philippines. Some of these rituals typically required the active participation of not only the patient but the patient's family and community members as well. Since ancient times, the cures for injuries and illness-causes mainly consisted of herbs, physical exercise, and fasts, all in combination with ritual. These were typical treatments in tribal medicine. Rituals were performed in which either the shaman and/or the patient performed an active role in the treatment.

In the introduction of Frank and Frank's (1991) book, *Persuasion and Healing,* third edition, the authors contend that the brain acts not only as the seat of consciousness, but also as the control mechanism for bodily functions, the nervous system, the endocrine system, and the immune system. "It also involves the way attitudes, moods, and emotions, processed by the brain, can promote health or set the stage for illness" (p. xi). Although the Franks' focus of healing principles is on psychotherapy, the authors address issues applicable to indigenous and CAM healing systems. "Examination of religious healing across cultures illuminates certain aspects of human functioning that are relevant to psychotherapy" (p. 87).

One conclusion of the authors was the importance of shifting the emphasis from differences in therapies to similarities. "The interaction between particular therapists and patients, determined by the personal qualities, values and expectations of both, contributes more to the outcome than does therapeutic technique" (1991, p. 300). The instillation of hope and anticipation of a positive outcome, the emotional arousal, and a sense of mastery are all brought about by the patient and healer taking active roles in the process of the healing. The healer's role incorporates acts of persuasion and includes the use of rhetoric. The three main factors prominent in effective healing experiences studied by Frank and Frank included hope or positive expectation, (b) emotional arousal, and (c) enhancement of the sense of mastery. The authors determined that patients who were most improved experienced improved mastery or felt more in control of their own life experience.

## The Torrey Model: Witchdoctors and Psychiatrists

E. F. Torrey, M. D., a clinical and research psychiatrist with a background in anthropology, published in 1972 *The Mind Game: Witchdoctors and Psychiatrists.* His revised book became *Witchdoctors and Psychiatrists: The Common Roots of Psychotherapy and its Future,* published in 1986. Torrey identified five fundamental principles operative in effective medicine, psychotherapy, and alternative healing systems. They include, first, that the healer's process of naming the affliction is the beginning of the therapeutic process. A shared worldview makes the diagnosing/ naming process possible (a precursor to the instillation of hope). Second, Torrey contends that specific personal qualities of the healer appear to facilitate recovery. These personal qualities include empathy, nonpossessive warmth, and personal genuineness. These are also the principles promoted by Carl Rogers (1957) as the essential elements in his client-centered therapy. Third, patient expectations of recovery assist in healing. Expectant faith, or the instillation of hope, was recognized by Sigmund Freud in 1940, and seems to positively affect healing processes. Torrey also concluded that the combination of the fourth principle (specific techniques) and the fifth (materials and healing procedures) empower the patient. Some healing rituals and materia medica used by indigenous healers are included in the results section of this study.

The Torrey model determines essential mechanisms of various systems of healing. These five essential elements that affect psychotherapy also seem to manifest, overlap, and blend with many of the other systems of healing frameworks employed by researchers. These principles apply not only to psychotherapy, but also provide a vehicle to transcend cultural barriers and are inclusive of indigenous healing practices and other alternative systems of healing. Torrey's model includes these five elements:

1. Patient expectations of healing.
2. A shared worldview.
3. The personal qualities of the healer.

4. Specific techniques.
5. Materials (materia medica).

These elements, combined with the healer's procedures, can assist in empowering the patient and promoting positive outcomes. This dynamic can be observed in shamanic healing ritual contexts. Taking an active role in one's own healing process can give a patient the sense of empowerment.

## Siegler and Osmond: Models of Madness and Medicine

Miriam Siegler, Ph.D., and Humphry Osmond, Ph.D. (1974), as have previous authors, took an innovative approach in investigating essential elements in both medical and psychiatric models of illness and healing, which may also apply to indigenous and CAM healing systems. Siegler and Osmond attempted to alleviate some confusion in the practice of medicine and psychiatry in the early 1970s by researching the various medical and psychiatric models prominent at that time. Their research grant was funded by the American Schizophrenic Foundation, founded in 1964. Siegler and Osmond presented the results of their research on conflicting medical and psychotherapeutic models in their 1974 book *Models of Madness, Models of Medicine.* Their emphasis on essential elements revealed that conflicts among the diverse models of illness and healing are prominent in the fields of medicine and psychiatry.

Siegler and Osmond contrasted eight models of medicine and psychotherapy:

1. Medical model.
2. Moral model.
3. Impaired model.
4. Psychoanalytic model.
5. Social model.
6. Psychedelic model.
7. Conspiratorial model.
8. Family interaction model.

They contrasted these models along 12 dimensions. Their analysis demonstrated both similarities and differences among psychotherapeutic systems on the following dimensions:

1. Diagnosis.
2. Etiology.
3. Patient's role.
4. Treatment.
5. Prognosis.
6. Suicide and death.
7. Institution.
8. Personnel.
9. Patient's rights and duties.
10. Family's rights and duties.
11. Rights and duties of society.
12. The goal of the model.

Siegler and Osmond (1974) also made comparisons between seven different alternative healing systems and the allopathic model. They pointed out that, within the allopathic model, the report of the patient's experience (symptoms) in combination with observation of the patient's behavior and examination of the patient's body (signs) can assist the diagnostic process. Treatment of signs and symptoms frequently proceeds in the absence of a known etiology. The diagnosis may be determined by trial and error. The treatment is oriented to a specific goal and is monitored by the response of the patient. Interventions may be chemical or procedural. Prognosis is based on the diagnosis and limits the possible outcomes. Within the allopathic model, death is seen as a failure of treatment, aging, or the inevitable result of a serious disease. But that is not necessarily so in other indigenous and CAM modes of treatment. For example, the Filipino espiritistas' diagnoses are not a process of trial and error, but are revealed to them by the Holy Spirit. The espiritistas believe in reincarnation and do not perceive death to be a finite failure of treatment.

Siegler and Osmond's framework has been utilized in studying complementary and alternative healing paradigms. They identified essential elements of illness and healing, including the roles of the patients and healers. They perceived that the patient's role involved certain privileges, yet it also involved limitations. For example, patients are exempt from ordinary responsibilities, but they have the duty to obey the healer. Siegler and Osmond also addressed the family's role. They were thorough in their investigation and the subsequent comparisons of various models and systems of healing. These essential elements affect patient role expectations and, therefore, affect individuals' illness and healing experiences. It appears that the NIHCAM panel elaborated on Siegler and Osmond's framework in developing the parameters for defining and describing complementary and alternative healing systems.

## The Parameters for Complementary and Alternative Medicine

In 1995, the U.S. National Institutes of Health Office ofAlternative Medicine sponsored a methodology conference in Bethesda, Maryland, and formed a committee to discuss complementary and alternative medicine (CAM). A variety of experts came together to attempt a new understanding of CAM that would be practical and inclusive. The parameters they created were to be used as a framework for understanding and classifying, in a new way, the great proliferation of alternative medical practices, both in the United States and elsewhere. The committee's work was the first attempt made by a Western agency in this field. The results of their efforts were subsequently published in the journal *Alternative Therapies in Health and Medicine* in the article, "Defining and Describing Complementary and Alternative Medicine" (O'Connor et al., 1997). The panel proposed a set of descriptive parameters for the qualitative research of complementary and alternative healing systems, which also represents a system of healing model. These parameters include the general categories of: (a) lexicon; (b) taxonomy; (c) epistemology; (d) theories; (e) goals for interventions; (f) outcome measures; (g) social organization; (h) specific activities and materials (materia medica); (i) responsibilities (patients, family, healer); U) scope; (k) analysis, benefits and barriers; (I) accommodation and view of suffering and death, and (m) comparison and interaction with more dominant systems. These parameters are broken down with more specific questions within each category (see appendix A).

A close look at the parameters generated by the conference and set forth by O'Connor et al. elucidates the inclusion of the aforementioned essential elements of systems of healing. Many of these concepts regarding illness and healing experiences had already been accepted by social workers and in public health medicine for several decades. According to O'Connor et al., theories need not be proposed to explain why an alternative healing system produces positive results. The only explanations necessary are those explanations provided by the practitioners themselves, from within the practitioner's own perspective. For example, the Filipino psychic surgeons report that their healing power is the Holy Spirit of God. This explanation is acceptable to the Filipino patients and practitioners and, therefore, is congruent with the CAM parameters in the description of a healing system.

The CAM parameters were presented to the National Institutes of Health Office of Alternative Medicine as a standard for inquiry and description. The detailed categories and in-depth questions from CAM provided the framework for describing a system of healing where formal theories need not be proposed to explain given outcomes in alternative healing methods. The open-ended nature of the CAM parameters makes it possible in the present study to make a comprehensive qualitative inquiry according to individual cultural definitions. The CAM parameters facilitate a richly detailed description of the system of healing used by the psychic surgeons in the Philippines.

While using the CAM parameters, it became apparent that some systems of healing defy classification per se. There are cross-cultural overlaps, use of multiple healing methods, spiritual involvement, and the occurrence of culturally influenced metaphysical events. The CAM parameters ask few questions specific to this uncharted area. The CAM parameters, having been forged as a tool to apply in domestic medical practice, and to enable health insurance companies to deal with the burgeoning of alternative medicine, could not be so inclusive as to include faith healing, sorcery, or psychic surgery. Hence, there are limitations when using the CAM parameters as a framework to describe the system of healing as used by the espiritistas in the Philippines.

The CAM parameters include many specific detailed questions regarding the breadth of the healing experience and cultural components. An astute reader will keep in mind, however, the source and function of the CAM parameters, no matter how inclusive they seem, because, as is said, consider the source. The U. S. government and its subcommittees, while dedicated to providing for the inclusion of alternative medicine into the giant health care industry, is still extremely skeptical of that which is difficult to describe, measure, and quantify, and it exhibits a genuine distaste for any medical system bordering on the paranormal. A truly postmodern approach would attempt to transcend political, geographic, and cultural borders altogether, thereby, allowing room for "medicine on the margin" (V. Thielen, personal communication, August 18, 2002).

## Krippner and Remen: Systems of Healing

Krippner and Remen (2000) summarized the previously mentioned researchers' findings and developed a model for a "systems of healing" university course, based on researchers' perceived essential elements of illness and healing experiences. Krippner and Remen presented a model for describing systems of healing consisting of these categories: (a) the illness, (b) the healer, the healing relationship, (d) the healing transaction, (e) the social issues, and (f) the ethical issues. Specific questions were proposed to assist in developing a description of a healing system.

Krippner and Remen also formulated a grid listing four essential healing principles. Placed on the horizontal axis are: (a) shared worldview, (b) personal qualities of the healer, (c) patient expectations, and (d) techniques and procedures. And there are five common factors in healing on the vertical axis: (a) the nature of the ailment, (b) nature of the patient, (c) nature of the environment, nature of the treatment, and (e) interactive factors. This grid exemplifies the variables affecting human beings' illnesses and healing experiences (Appendix B).

Krippner and Remen contended that, regardless of which model one uses, several essential healing principles will persist. The universal principles are: (a) naming the ailment, (b) patient's expectancy and attitude, (c) the nature of the environment (e.g., family, friends, and community), (d) the nature of the treatment, and (e) the interactions of these factors. The elements affected by human consciousness, which emerge and which require further research, are placebo or expectancy effects and the patient-healer relationship. Many writers and researchers have contributed to this emerging body of thought. The system of healing approach is the overarching method used to describe the relationships between patient, healer, and cure.

Researchers and medical scientists have worked diligently for many generations to try to describe, define, and classify illnesses and diseases as to cause and cure. The results of biomedical research are overwhelming in the depth of detail and usefulness as diagnostic tools. Such research has yielded great authority and a firmness of belief in its classifications, which supposedly rivals no other. The biomedical system of classification and prescribed methods of healing are also always changing as new information is accumulated. Yet, the biomedical model does not generally allow for the integration of information outside of the empirical perspective.

## Applying the Archival Data to the Systems of Healing Models

Evaluations by the systems of healing theorists suggest that the CAM parameters are a basis of establishing completeness according to the essential principles of the proposed healing system. There are many other systems of healing besides those practiced by the Western mainstream. As a new theoretical framework, the systems of healing approach acknowledges different definitions of illness and health across cultures, some of which acknowledge the plurality of meanings. While using some of the same classifications of diseases, the systems of healing approach takes into account human consciousness, the individual and societal experience of illness and healing, factors of unique cultures, personal awareness, and the social environment.

The firsthand observations and secondary reports of psychic surgery (as well as accounts by the healers themselves) have been applied to the CAM parameters. The CAM parameters' format for description controlled for both discipline and personal bias. Applying the systems of healing approach as a research method has distinct advantages for this study. Remaining questions are: (a) What data are there to support the claims? (b) What data appear to refute the claims? and (c) How can additional research be accomplished?

The CAM parameters for alternative medicine provide the framework for the inquiry and description of the many facets of the healing practices of the espiritistas and act as an invaluable model. Fundamental questions are addressed by the systems of healing approach. The systems of healing approach allows for great latitude in defining illness and for answering what types of treatment are appropriate. If the experience of illness is culture-bound, so also are the methods used to heal. "We might not use herbs and spells to heal a broken ankle in California, but the same remedy might be completely appropriate for a depressed person in rural Philippines" (V. Thielen, personal communication, August 18, 2002).

# VI RESULTS

When the National Institutes of Health Office of Alternative Medicine recognized the need to formally address the issues of alternative medicine, a committee was formed for this special purpose. Among the research, activities, and recommendations performed by the committee was the creation of a set of guidelines to be used for the definition and understanding of alternative health systems; the document is known as *The Parameters for Description of Complementary and Alternative Medicine.* The following results section is the literature and archival data collected during this study of the Filipino Espiritistas' system of healing applied to that set of parameters.

## The Parameters for Description of Complementary and Alternative Medicine

### *Lexicon*

### What Are the Specialized Terms in the System?

*Espiritistas.* Espiritistas is a term of Spanish/Philippine origin, meaning persons who have the ability to channel the spiritual energy of, or be possessed by, the Holy Spirit for positive healing goals. "What Filipinos call faith healers and psychic surgeons may be classified as spiritual healers [espiritistas]" (Licauco, 1977, p. 15). Espiritistas are able to perform spiritual and magnetic healing, and most notably in the Philippines, psychic surgery. Espiritistas claim to have special relationships with the Holy Spirit and with the spirit world of discarnate entities, which they are able to contact to achieve a healing experience on the physical plane. Espiritistas or spiritual healers in most classification systems are synonymous with mediums. Mediums and spiritual healers believe that their actions are inspired or actually performed by spiritual energies.

*Christian Spiritism.* Christian Spiritism is a specialized clustering of religious/philosophical orientations arising from the combination of traditional Christianity with the more esoteric and paranormal notions of the Spiritist movement from the turn of the century influenced by Allen Kardec.

> Christian Spiritism is an interpretation of Christian doctrine that emphasizes the role of the Holy Spirit. Spiritism in the Philippines originally derived from the amalgamation of Christianity and pre existing shamanic and animistic beliefs. Christian Spiritism was reformulated by the Filipinos along lines of the philosophy of the French spiritualist Allen Kardec. (Martin, 1998, p. 244)

The Union of Espiritistas of the Philippines is a religious organization founded for the purpose of training gifted healers to become espiritistas and to gather its congregation in rituals of union with the Holy Spirit (Martin, 1998). This spiritual amalgam exhibits cultural specificity, but it is not limited to the Philippine Islands. Infused with the most intense beliefs in the Holy Spirit of God and the powers of healing referred to in the Bible, with its plethora of saints, devout Christians who were concurrently exposed to belief in the possibility of contacting spirits and discarnate entities often became so aroused as to be able to exhibit extraordinary powers, allegedly channeling the voice of God's Holy Spirit and allegedly perform healing miracles such as those referred to in the Bible. "Here, in the Philippines, the forces of Christ in the spirit world made themselves manifest through our mediums" (Alvear, cited in Martin, 2000a, p. 8). The Holy Spirit is perceived as a potent healing power and utilizes the medium for purposes of healing or the transmission of messages to the physical world.

*Magnetic healing.* Magnetic energy is described as the universal force that causes matter to form bonds or to disperse. It is the vital energy (*prana* in Sanskrit or *bisa* in Tagalog) that infuses all things. To possess wisdom of this vital magnetic energy is an ancient source of spiritual knowledge in nearly all cultures. The field of magnetic energy surrounds all objects and beings, and it radiates out in all directions. It is believed that disturbances in the flow of the magnetic field may cause illness, and it becomes the healer's task to tap into the stream of magnetic energy and effect a rebalance. According to Licauco (1977),

> Pranic or magnetic healing is a form in which the healer sends a supply of prana (also called odic-force, animal magnetism and orgone energy) to the affected parts of the patient, thus stimulating the cells and tissues to normal activity and ejecting waste matter from the body. Magnetic healing is normally accomplished by either passing or laying of hands on the affected patient. This is a universal practice that dates back to ancient history. Magnetic healing works because it induces changes in the physical body by altering the flow of vitality at the subtle etheric levels of man's constitution. (pp. 7-8)

Magnetic healing is the method by which an individual of reputed high spiritual sensibilities may be able to consciously induce trance states to skillfully manipulate the subtle vital force of electromagnetism. The technique requires both the power of concentration of the healer in his own union with this energy and the ability to focus it on another person, in order to make substantial changes on the physical plane. "Laying on of hands" is the healer's method of manipulating magnetism to direct energy for the relief of depleted areas. The Filipino espiritistas perceive this power to be the Holy Spirit of God. Donald McDowall (1998) reports on magnetic healing:

> Magnetic healing had the same effects as psychic surgery, but the technique was different, he [Jun Labo] said, "Magnetic healing melts the condition. If there is cancer, magnetic healing will melt this." The hands had to be kept moving to keep the current flowing. Magnetic healing was a laying on of hands. (pp. 94-95)

*Psychic Surgery.* Psychic surgery is a specialized modality or subset of spiritual healing, allegedly conducted by using the bare hands to enter the body, extracting tumors or other obstructions, while the patient is conscious, without pain or the use of anesthetic, leaving no scars or only minimal scaring. Psychic surgery is a direct application of the major phenomenon of mediumship. The healer acts as a medium, or channel, for spiritual and magnetic energies to flow through himself and into the patient. By means of the skill in manipulating magnetic energy, the healer is able to penetrate the body-both the spiritual body and the physical body. Alex Orbito explained psychic surgery to Harvey Martin (1998):

> When my spiritual mind is attuned to the Holy Spirit of God, my hand emits an energy that is more powerful than the physical makeup of the human cells, which merely give way to a more powerful force. When I put my hand inside the body, my hand is like a magnet. So, even if the sickness is a distance from my hand, it is drawn to me and I feel a current. When I feel the current, I know the sickness is now in my hand and I remove it immediately. (pp. 18-19)

The espiritistas claim that some psychic surgery is spirit directed while other surgeries may be therapeutic sleight-of-hand (Martin, 1998). Minor surgeries are performed without anesthetic or antibiotics. The espiritistas claim that, during their operations, the Holy Spirit acts as an anesthetic and antibiotic while controlling the loss of blood. Although Alvear incorporated the Union of Espiritistas of the Philippines in 1909, and the church began openly practicing mediumship trainings, it was not until 1948 that the technique of spirit-directed psychic surgery was utilized by the Filipino Kardec influenced espiritistas.

It is reported by Licauco (1999) and others that Eluterio Terte was performing magnetic healing on a patient, when he looked down to discover that the patient's body had opened up, and his hands were inside the patient's body. He became nervous but allowed the Spirit to continue to direct his hands, as it was the Holy Spirit, not himself, who was actually performing the operation. These were additions of new techniques to the Union of Espiritistas' treatment modalities: minor surgery, spirit-directed psychic surgery, and therapeutic sleight-of-hand psychic surgery. It is reported by Martin (1998) and others that when the espiritistas were performing magnetic healing on individuals while under the influence of the Holy Spirit, several espiritistas spontaneously began to perform psychic surgeries.

There are many references to anomalous healings achieved through the practice of mediumship, combining the energies of the Spirit, the medium or espiritista, and the patient (Licauco, 1999, Martin, 1998; McDowall, 1998). The restoration of health through spirit-directed psychic surgeries is not specifically identified in *A Short Spiritist Doctrine,* Alvear's book written in 1909 (cited in Martin 2000a). It is only suggested that the espiritistas, while in spirit directed trance, refer to "miraculous" forms of healing as referred to in the Bible. Some espiritistas refer to the practice of spirit-directed psychic surgery as a spiritual operation (Martin, 2002b). They have adopted the Western term to some degree. *Psychic surgery* was a term coined by Harold Sherman (1966), a Westerner who observed these interventions practiced by espiritistas in Brazil and the Philippines.

*Witchcraft (Kulam).* Practices of witchcraft *(kulam)* include the use of personal power, spirits, or demons to inflict harm on others, usually causing physical, spiritual, or psychological distress. Whereas Lieban (1967) makes a distinction between sorcerers *(mangkukulam)* and witches *(aswang)* in the Visayas in Northern Luzon, the espiritistas (when explaining these illnesses to Westerners) simply refer to the illnesses as the results of witchcraft. "The witchcraft cult that exists in the Philippines is ancient and powerful" (Martin, 1998, p. 29). Filipinos frequently regard witchcraft *(kulam)* or sorcery *(panggagaway)* as causes of both illness and misfortune. Witchcraft *(kulam)* can also be described as malign activities, including those of spirits and human beings capable of harming others through the use of supernatural power. When a person has been influenced by a hex or spell *(buyag),* that person may become ill in any variety of ways. One of the most common acts of sorcery in the Visayas is *barang,* sending bugs, rocks, broken glass, or other foreign objects into the body of the intended victim (Lieban, 1967, p. 65).

## How Are Common Health and Illness Terms Distinctively Defined by the System?

According to the Filipino espiritistas' system of healing, one is determined to be in good health *(kalusugan)* when engaged in a process of spiritual *(banal)* development. Health is not only freedom from physical symptoms, but also the maintenance of spiritual *(banal)* balance and growth. Illness *(sakit)*, on the other hand, may be the result of sorcery or a negative physical manifestation resulting from acts of sin (sa/a) or from a sinful lifestyle. Illness in the Philippines can also result from becoming a victim *(biktima)* of malign magic, witchcraft *(gayuma)*, or sorcery *(panggagaway)*. Other unnatural or metaphysical events influenced by nature spirits *(enkantos)* or other spiritual beings can also result in illness experiences. The espiritistas refer to these metaphysical conditions as simply "witchcraft" due to the linguistic, cultural, and conceptual barriers that exist in translating these complex concepts for most Westerners.

## What Are the Terms Used to Identify Roles and People Within the System?

The espiritistas believe that they act as mediums of the Holy Spirit to perform healing on patients. Mediums, who believe they are blessed with the healing gift, utilize techniques of magnetic healing or other traditional healing methods. The more dynamic healers supposedly are gifted with the ability to perform spirit directed minor surgeries or therapeutic sleight-of-hand psychic surgeries. Espiritistas, tambalans, or mananambal all purport to provide healing within the spiritual and physical realms.

Patients *(pasyente)* come to espiritistas for diverse ailments and distress. Many Filipinos prefer the local practitioners to Western trained biomedical practitioners due to the shared worldview, affordability, and convenience. Patients generally experience trust and have faith in the activities of their indigenous healers.

Sorcerers *(mangkukulam)* or witches *(aswang)* who utilize malign magic to affect individuals, supposedly, are often the cause of illness experienced by patients. Patients are often concerned they may mistakenly visit a sorcerer while seeking treatment from tambalans or mananambal. Sorcery is one of human beings' earliest explanations for illness, disease, bad luck, bad fate, or otherwise unexplainable events.

## Taxonomy

## What Classes of Health and Illness or Disease Does the System Recognize and Address?

Health *(kalusugan)* and illness *(sakit)* categories are easily described in this healing system. The patients (pasyente) come to the espiritistas for both natural *(likas)* and unnatural *(di-kilala)* ailments. Natural *(likas)* ailments are medically diagnosable conditions, and an ailment is considered unnatural *(di-ki/ala)* when a medical condition cannot be determined. Natural or physical illnesses may be consistent with Western biomedical diagnoses.

> The Luzon healers are particularly adept at dealing with diseased tissue, blood clots, and [infections]. I have seen them remove an appendix, excise growths from the breast, open cysts, shrink bladder stones, varicose veins and hemorrhoids, and even treat several types of cancer with excellent results. (Watson, 1974, p. 219)

Illnesses may be classified as unnatural maladies when the condition is caused by sin, witchcraft, or sorcery. In Luzon, espiritistas will oftentimes diagnose a person's problem as being caused by witchcraft (whereas in the Visayas, the cause of the illness is referred to as sorcery). The psychic surgeon may then proceed to remove foreign objects from the patient's body, such as rope, rocks, or leaves, and miscellaneous substances. The espiritistas claim they do not know what form the negative energy will take while being removed from the patient's body. Spiritual illnesses can manifest in many different forms. These surgeries are frequently documented in the writings from the earliest accounts until present. Valentine (1973) reports an account of a patient who was a witchcraft victim (mangkukulam biktima):

> The girl was not in pain, but she was evidently upset at the thought of being a witchcraft victim. Suddenly several large, flat leaves from some tropical plant popped up from the surgical opening like a jack-in-the-box. I stared in blank disbelief as the crowd behind me gasped in unison. Mercado plucked the leaves out of the girl and waved them to the onlookers. (pp. 102-103)

Nearly all types of spiritual imbalances and physical ailments are treated by the espiritistas.

## What Causes for Illness Does the System Recognize?

The espiritistas recognize both natural and unnatural causes of illness. The espiritistas believe acts of sin, a sinful lifestyle, or the imposition of witchcraft/sorcery all can create negative energy within the body that may lead to physical illness. Sin is a very general term that can include a vast array of thoughts and behaviors. Broadly, sin can be conceptualized as those thoughts and behaviors that separate the individual from God and, therefore, result in natural illnesses. It is perceived that true human nature is to be at one with, or in communion with, God in thought, word, and deed. This state of righteous union results in the experience of wellness or good health. According to Orbito (cited in Martin, 1998, p. 27), occasionally God will allow illness as an educational experience for an individual who needs to learn lessons of compassion and humility. Premature death is viewed as God's decision for a soul to transition to the spiritual world.

The other explanation for unnatural illness is simply witchcraft. The espiritistas in the Visayas more often perceive sorcery to be the unnatural cause of illness. Imbalances of *bisa,* or vital energy, and manifestations of negative forces are sometimes perceived as the result of witchcraft and are recognized as major causes of illness. Physical manifestations of illness in the body can be treated utilizing the healing and balancing of magnetic energy, *bisa,* or the Holy Spirit. This negative energy of necessity affects biological tissues, giving rise to illness. Damaged organs and tissues; tumors, cancerous or benign; and cartilage and calcium deposits are all treated by the use of magnetic healing or psychic surgery.

## How Important Is It to Identify and Address Ultimate, as Opposed to Proximate, Causes of Illness?

The ultimate or proximate causes of illnesses do not appear to be of any great significance to the espiritistas. However, if the illness is acute and requires an immediate intervention, such as magnetic healing or psychic surgery, the espiritistas will initially diagnose for witchcraft prior to performing any treatment.

Sin, a sinful lifestyle, witchcraft, or sorcery are generally considered to be the ultimate causes of illness, which can result in physical manifestations of negative or blocked energies and may result in organ-specific illnesses. The physical results of blocked energies can oftentimes be diagnosed with Western medicine and may be considered the proximate cause.

Illnesses caused by witchcraft cannot be diagnosed or successfully treated with the use of Western medicine. Illness resulting from witchcraft or sorcery must be treated by an espiritista or tambalan. Any illness may manifest physically or remain in the spiritual realm, causing bad luck or bad fate. Espiritistas appear to treat organ-specific ailments with their special surgical procedures and, at the same time, treat spiritual maladies and spiritual perspectives on illness experiences.

## Epistemology

## Is There a Canonical Body of Knowledge?

The canonical body of knowledge embraced by the Union of Espiritistas is found in the treatise *A Short Spiritist Doctrine*. Juan Alvear, a highly educated and articulate man who was also a healer, founded the Union of Espiritistas of the Philippines on January 21, 1909, and wrote the first text of the Union of Espiritistas Church *(A Short Spiritist Doctrine,)* which was translated into English by Siegfried Sepulveda and later published by Harvey Martin in 2000. The cover page of Martin's edition includes the statement, "Adapted from the writings of the first apostle of Spiritism, Allen Kardec, and the result of thorough research by the author on true spiritism" (Martin, 1998, p. 68).

Kardec had published his first book on spiritism in 1857, titled *The Spirit's Book*. In this book, he and two mediums asked 1,018 questions of spirit entities. The spirits answered questions on the topics of primary causes; the spiritual world; moral, natural, and divine law; and repentance, purgatory, and hell, according to early translations. According to Alvear's (1909) *A Short Spiritist's Doctrine* (cited in Martin, 2000a), the use of psychic surgery is the Holy Spirit making itself known to the physical world, in order to promote belief in God and to further the spiritual progress of humankind. Psychic surgeons proclaim that the power of the Holy Spirit has brought worldwide attention to the Philippines and the espiritistas through their healing practices. This postulate is congruent with the claims made by *A Short Spiritist's Doctrine*. Martin (1998) refers to the Kardec spiritist communities:

> The spiritist communities of Brazil and the Philippines share the unusual distinction of practicing very similar methods of paranormal healing within the gospel message of Jesus' healing ministry. These traditions of spirit-directed healing, when articulated by the spiritual revelations in the books of Allan Kardec, and applied within the context of the miraculous healing ministry of Jesus, produced (a set of practices) in which psychic surgery has emerged as one of the primary modes of treatment. (p. 74)

## How Do the Origins and Social History of the System Relate to Current Theories and Practices?

Martin (1998) contends that, "Since ancient times, the Filipinos have possessed a highly sophisticated understanding of the inner working of the spiritual realm, as well as the different types of supernatural power through which healing is accomplished" (p. 53). Written documentation of the Filipinos' early indigenous healing practices are nearly nonexistent. What is known is that their early practices were similar to other Southeast Asian shamanistic practices (Heinze, 1997; Winkelman, 1992). Filipinos have a long history of spiritual contact, negotiation, and spiritual or metaphysical warfare (hexes, etc.) prior to the arrival of the Spanish. Upon the introduction of Spanish Catholicism, native Filipinos experienced an absence of conceptual conflicts with their own belief systems, and the Holy Spirit was accepted as the mediator between themselves and God (Licauco, 1999, Martin, 1998).

Filipinos were once completely dependent on folk medicine for diagnosis and treatment of illnesses, including those illnesses attributed to sorcery. Even with a marked increase of Western trained practitioners who do not accept magical explanations of disease, notions about sorcery are substantially the same after 4 centuries, in spite of significant changes in other aspects of Cebuano life. Acts of sorcery were prevalent in the pre-Christian era, in times when the manananbal called on nature spirits for their power. According to Martin (1998) Christianity contained elements which, to many Filipinos, appeared to be a highly developed form of spirit-directed healing and exorcism and provided the manananbal with fertile ground for incorporating their own ancient system of shamanism into Christianity.

The Union of Espiritistas of the Philippines embraces the practice of spiritism and, primarily, the healing methods of magnetic healing and psychic surgery. The Union of Espiritistas of the Philippines continues with its original theoretical principles of mediumship for the purpose of healing, incorporating Allen Kardec's concepts, which were introduced to the Philippine community by Juan Alvear, the founder of Christian spiritism. Mediumship trainings are necessary to become an espiritista, and training begins with studying the Holy Scriptures, as well as engaging in the worship of God.

The Bible frequently mentions the act of God putting words into the mouths of the prophets. It is interpreted from the Book of Acts that the apostles were filled with the outpouring of the Holy Spirit, and that the apostles were actually experiencing possession by the Holy Spirit of God. Kardec and his followers, over the decades, interpreted this occurrence as an example of mediumship. Other phenomena that may take place during trance states are mentioned in the Bible: spirit writing, hearing spirits, seeing spirits, and spirit communication in dreams.

During the church services of the Union Espiritistas of the Philippines, it is believed the Holy Spirit delivers sermons through mediums in trance. The mediums perform automatic writing with references to the scriptures, as the Spirit channels the message through them. The Holy Spirit also channels messages through a medium who operates an apparatus (known as a ouija board in the West), which is best described as a circular board with the letters of the alphabet and the numbers 1 through 10 printed on it, set up on a tripod. The medium operates the apparatus as the spirit allegedly answers questions by spelling out words and revealing numbers (Martin, 1998, p. 128).

According to Kardec, Alvear, and others, the gifts of the Holy Spirit are divided into three categories:
1. The gifts of Revelation, which include words of wisdom, words of knowledge, and discernment of the true spirit.
2. The gifts of Power, which include the gift of faith, the gift of healing, and the gift of working miracles.
3. The gifts of Inspiration, which include the gift of prophesy, the gift of diversity of tongues, and the interpretation of languages bestowed with these gifts of the Holy Spirit.

Also important to the espiritistas are the examples of Jesus working as an instrument of Holy Spirit. His first instruction to the apostles was to "heal the sick, cleanse the lepers, and cast out demons." A medium, also working with the Holy Spirit, can heal by placing his hands on the body of an ill person; in other cases, the medium can heal by only looking at the afflicted part or, simply, the sickness will be cured by the presence of the medium.

## What Are the Internal Disputes and Variables of the System?

In the early days of the Union, most practices were based on the teachings of Christ, which created internal cohesion. In Allan Kardec's book *The Gospel: Explained by the Spiritist Doctrine* (2000, translated from the 1866 3rd ed.), he disputed the virgin birth, the crucifixion, and the resurrection of Jesus Christ. These notions were always unpopular in the Philippines, even though Christian spiritism or "true spiritism" flourished. The mid 1960s exposed many Union members to different spiritual beliefs and practices, and many members wanted to abandon Christian Spiritism to form a nondenominational fraternity of mediums. Many members no longer wanted the Union to be defined as Christian Spiritism. The emerging popularity of psychical research seemed, for many, a more appropriate way to explain the mysteries inherent in Spiritism. One of the prominent espiritistas, Terte, resigned from the Union of Espiritistas of the Philippines and incorporated The Christian Spiritists of the Philippines, Inc. in 1955. About 40% of the Union members remained with Terte. The others incorporated the influences of Western psychical notions and Eastern religions, thus, becoming a more nondenominational group of psychic healers (Martin, 1998, p. 26).

## How Does the System Respond to Novel Input?

Singer (1990) contends psychic surgeons made a transition from being traditional indigenous mediums, accessing the aid of nature spirits, to a "simulacrum of Western medicine" utilizing the more socially acceptable notion of the Holy Spirit, supposedly received in trance (p. 449). Filipinos' exposure to Western surgical methods had increased during the course of World War II. This increased exposure to Western surgical methods may have resulted in the new healing technique referred to as psychic surgery.

Many of the Filipino espiritistas responded positively to the introduction of psychical research and input from the discipline of parapsychology. The practice of psychic surgery centered on a strong form of spirit-directed medicine, yet these new philosophies had much to offer in expanding an understanding of their healing system. There were no major conflicts with the concept of psychic healing and their existing spiritual healing practices, although there has been little assimilation of other practices.

A growing community of believers, followers, and practitioners of psychic surgery and other healing methods accepted psychic explanations for the phenomena using insights from the realms of quantum physics, psychokinesis, ectoplasmic formations, materializations, and teleportations. Many healers embraced concepts from the Far East, such as *karma, prana,* and *chakras* (Singer, 1990, p. 449), while others embraced theories regarding spiritual or bioplasmic bodies. In response to the increasing international input from alternative practitioners and other interested parties, Alex Orbito formed the Philippine Healers' Circle, Inc. in 1981. This organization, an international group of healers, accepted associate members from around the world in 1986, as they hosted the first Philippine International Healing Festival in Manila.

## Theories (Links to Taxonomy and Epistemology) What Are Important Human Systems, Their Mechanisms of Action, and Their Interconnections Understood to Be?

The espiritistas believe that the most important human systems are spiritual and physical. The mechanism of action of each is held to be largely the work of the Holy Spirit in the form of magnetic energy, or the vital force that manifests in the practice of mediumship or trance healing. Mediumship is purportedly one of the gifts of the so called energy of the Holy Spirit. The medium claims to develop the ability to direct the Holy Spirit's magnetic energy in the processes of magnetic healing and psychic surgery.

According to Alvear's *A Short Spiritist Doctrine* (Martin, 2000a), everyone has the ability to become a medium, although this skill needs to be developed. Supposedly, the gift of mediumship has been given to humanity by God to be used for good deeds and to help propagate the teaching of God. The members of The Union of Espiritistas of the Philippines practice the art and skill of mediumship. Elders of the church provide the instruction during mediumship trainings. It is believed that when one develops the ability to go into trance, the gifts of the Holy Spirit can be received.

Benjamin Pajarillo (cited in Martin, 1998) provides an excellent summary of a system of healing that incorporates spirituality into its healing practices. The Filipino espiritistas embrace Christian beliefs and a broad worldview in their spiritual practices. These "spiritual prerequisites," the special understanding and insight of healers, were further explained by Pajarillo. He promoted a spiritual prerequisite for the optimal effectiveness of all therapeutic interaction. One must first pray and concentrate that the will of God be done. "Second, one calls on the Holy Spirit to intervene, allowing the light of God to come and operate through both the healer and patient" (p. 141). The healer, with the aid of the Holy Spirit, makes a diagnosis and is directed by the Spirit with the proper course of treatment. These beliefs regarding trance healing include divine interventions within the healing acts. Understanding practitioners as instruments of the healing power of the Holy Spirit of God is said to remove the limitations of dualistic thought (p. 141).

According to Martin (1998), the Holy Spirit of God will direct energy to the afflicted area that needs to be healed. True mediumship healing is the power of both the Holy Spirit and the magnetic energy of the medium. The body of the espiritista is used to direct the mixed spiritual "fluids" into the body of the patient. The Holy Spirit vitalizes the afflicted patient with additional magnetic fluid, which the spirit produces by the exertion of its will. This impulsion of magnetic fluid, willed by the Holy Spirit, is directed through the body of the healer into the patient (p. 188).

According to *A Short Spiritist Doctrine* (Martin, 2000a), magnetism is a term used to describe universal power fluids. There are four main fluids. Magnetic fluid comes from the earth, from minerals, from vegetables, and from animals. The heat of the human body is also said to be good medicine. The animal "liquid" that emanates from the human body is curative in and of itself. When augmented by an elevated spirit, the healing is thought to be more effective. According to the espiritistas, this so-called magnetic energy facilitates the healing process. The healer need not exert effort, except to touch the patient with the hand. Objects held by the medium can be vehicles for curing: blessed oil, water, paper, a handkerchief, and so on, all of which can cure if they have been touched by a spirit medium. Martin (1998) states, "Through understanding and mastering these spiritual prerequisites as the primary means of healing, and fully integrating them into personal interaction with a patient, any and all forms of medicine can be instantly transformed into spirit-directed medicine" (pp. 141-142).

It is held that most of these healings are not possible without the help of the Blessed Spirit through the will of God. Kardec believed that mediums (espiritistas) who could communicate with the spiritual world could also utilize their abilities as healers.

> Kardec believed that the spirit is enveloped in a semi-material body of its own which he named the perispirit. The perispirit is composed of a magnetic fluid which contains a certain amount of electricity. It serves as an intermediary between one's spiritual body and physical body. Thus Kardec stated that healing can be accomplished by psychic healers who send magnetic rays from their fingertips into the auras of ill persons. By using these magnetic passes, a healer

can also magnetize water which can be used for healing purposes. "Healers" may sometimes be mediums and communicate with various spirits, [in Brazil and other spiritist communities] these entities are usually relatives, or distinguished people such as doctors, writers, and teachers. (Krippner & Villoldo, 1976, p. 119)

Kardec (cited in Krippner & Villoldo, 1976) claimed to receive information from spirits through mediums. His writings also include information that he said came to him directly from the spirit world. In *The Mediums' Book,* Kardec claimed that the medium acts as an intermediary between spirits and humans. The healing energy referred to as "fluid" is a magnetic force that belongs to humans, "yet its power is enhanced through the aid of spirits" (p. 123). There are healers around who do not credit spirits. Yet the spirits do not assist only those who believe in them. "Anyone who magnetizes for a good purpose is calling the spirits without being aware of it" (p. 123).

## How Are the Symptoms Interpreted Within the System, Generally and Specifically?

Symptoms of discomfort, physical ailments, and illnesses are generally perceived as the manifestations of sin or a sinful lifestyle. Sin is said to result in spiritual imbalance. Spiritual imbalance then results in physical symptoms. Specifically, the espiritistas acknowledge the symptoms and causes of most Western biomedical diagnoses (e.g., cancer, high blood pressure, diabetes, liver disease) as treatable with the use of their spiritual methods. All illnesses are perceived to exist in both the spiritual and physical realms. Therefore, interventions or treatments can be provided in either realm.

Occasionally the effects of sorcery or witchcraft (malign magic) are blamed for illness experiences. Espiritistas may diagnose witchcraft or sorcery and remove objects resulting from the malign magic from the victim's body. Agpaoa (as cited in Martin 2002b) commented on the notion that God punishes people through the use of illness experiences:

Many people suppose that God sends sickness because the Lord in His mysterious providence willed for them to be sick. Some believe that the Lord regularly Punishes his children through sickness. Though it is true that God sometimes permits sickness to come as a matter of discipline, He does not punish man with sickness except in the most flagrant cases. (p. 32)

## What Is the Relationship of Preventative and Therapeutic Actions to Illness and Prevention or Melioration of Illness?

The Filipino espiritistas perceive spiritual growth and the worship of God as the best preventative measures and believe these practices will generally prevent the experience of illnesses. According to Orbito (as cited in Martin, 1998):

If your physical body is not balanced, when you come in contact with illness or diseases, it will have a negative influence on you. That is why you must balance your body with your meditation and prayer so that the sickness will disappear through your sincerity to God. (p. 16)

Faith in God is essential for both the prevention of illness, as well as the healing process. It is believed that refraining from sinful acts and living in accordance with God's word is necessary to maintain both spiritual and physical health. 'The espiritistas often tell their patients that faith in God and the surrender to the will of God are the most important factors in the restoration of health" (Martin, 1998, p. 27).

## What Is the Role of Patients' Beliefs or Expectations of Practitioners' Intent?

The patient's faith and belief about the practitioner's intention are held to be critical to successful interventions. The patient's spiritual growth is always central to maintain health. While Orbito claims the patient's belief in God is not absolutely necessary for an initial intervention to take place, there must be a minimal expectation that the healer has special abilities. Initial interventions can take place irrespective of the patient's belief in the system. Agpaoa says his patients heal themselves. "I merely plant the seed with my surgery; the patient's mind does the rest" (Martin, 2002b, p. 2). Agpaoa addresses the topic of faith in *The Gifts of the Spirit:*

> To one He [Jesus Christ] said, 'Thy faith has made thee whole." To another He said, "According to your faith be it unto you. If thou canst believe all things are possible to him that believith" (Mark 9:23). To the invalid who was helpless for thirty-eight years He said, "Wilt thou be made whole?" It is notable that Christ did not usually heal the person who came for deliverance until He had first given him some instruction. "Faith cometh by hearing, and hearing by the word of God" (Romans, 10:17). (p. 40)

Psychic surgery is believed to be a demonstration of the power of the Holy Spirit, and the experience will hopefully inspire patients in their belief. According to the espiritistas, the ailment may return if the patients do not pursue their spiritual development. During the initial healing transaction, the role of the patients is to repent for their sins, to remove sinful thoughts, and to request forgiveness for those behaviors that have separated them from God. Then the Holy Spirit can perform a healing process upon the patients.

## Goals for Interventions

## What Are the Primary Goals of the System?

The goals of this system are not only the successful treatment of physical ailments, but they also include the treatment of spiritual illnesses, including malign human agency or witchcraft, to promote wellness and peace of mind, to encourage belief in God, and to assist the development of patients' spiritual growth. According to Kardec's followers and many of the Filipino espiritistas, the Holy Spirit is making itself known to the physical world through the practice of psychic surgery and other events taking place during the practice of mediumship.

## Outcome Measures

## What Constitutes a Successful Intervention?

The balancing of magnetic energy in the body and the dissolving or removal of diseased tissues or foreign matter from the body are both considered successful surgical interventions. According to Martin (1998)

> The restoration of health is a real, measurable experience. To receive the gift of restored health, restored life, directly from God, is a profound and transformational event. Spirit-directed restoration of health can become a bonding experience with God when it takes place in a supportive environment. (p. 156)

These successful interventions result in a remission of symptoms, induction or a restoration of faith, peace of mind, removal of a hex or curse, a restoration of balance and harmony, and revitalization of weak or suppressed vital energy according to the Filipino espiritistas' system of healing.

## How Are Successful Interventions Evaluated?

Word of mouth or personal testimonies are the only evaluations made within this healing system, and, to be contextually sensitive, these should not be evaluated according to the Western biomedical perspective. Previous scientific testing proved inconclusive or provided conflicting information regarding blood and tissue samples from psychic surgeries. For as many allegations of fraud, there have been numerous testimonies of successful healing (Licauco, 1999; Martin, 1998, 1999; McDowall, 1998; Sherman, 1966; Stelter, 1976; Valentine, 1973).

The Filipinos' system of healing requires alternative approaches of inquiry to evaluate what exactly can be considered the restoration of health or positive outcomes from specific interventions. Successful outcomes may include remission of symptoms, induction or restoration of faith, peace of mind, removal of a hex or curse, a restoration of balance and harmony, and/or revitalization of weak or suppressed vital energy.

## How Are the Successes and Failures of Treatments and Practitioners Explained?

The successes of the Philippine faith healers and psychic surgeons are attributed to the glory of God and the healing capacity of the Holy Spirit. Martin (1998) emphasizes the importance of faith in the healing experience. He reports that many times the healers would advise their patients to pray, meditate, and surrender to God. Patients sometimes would ignore this advice, clinging to the idea that the healer alone possessed the power to heal them, in spite of everything that the healers tell them. This dynamic can become a particular concern when the patient is not healed. The healer will receive the blame for the patient not being cured. "It is much easier to blame the healer than it is to blame God, ourselves, or fate" (p. 27). According to the healers, failures to heal are attributed to God's will, to fate, and the failure of the patients to continue with their spiritual growth and development, a belief which can neither be proven nor falsified by research.

## Social Organization
## What Are the Prevalence and Distribution of This System?

The Philippine province of Pangasinan (approximately a 1- day bus ride North of Manilla) in Northern Luzon is considered the heartland of Christian Spiritism. The actual number of healers who practice psychic surgery is undetermined, although Pangasinan is where the practice of psychic surgery is most prevalent. Many healers have established practices in Baugio City and Manila, and at least one member of the Union, Emilio Laporga, has established a practice much further south in Cebu City. Espiritistas have traveled to the United States, Europe, South America, and elsewhere. However, the difficulties of traveling challenge the practitioner's physical and spiritual balance, oftentimes negatively affecting their healing abilities. The mananambal and tambalans are indigenous healers, some of whom utilize trance healing or mediumship, which qualify them as espiritistas. These practitioners are spread throughout the lower regions in the Philippine Islands, the Visyas, and Mindanao.

## Who Uses the System or to Whom Is It Particularly Accessible?

Local Filipinos and some foreigners are inclined to pursue alternative medicine and utilize this healing system. The espiritistas are easily accessible to the local Filipinos, whereas foreigners have to travel a great distance, which is sometimes difficult for people who are experiencing illness (Nolen, 1974). Often those patients who have been given a poor prognosis from allopathic practitioners will travel to the Philippines as a last effort to restore their health. In rare occurrences, people in other countries have utilized psychic surgeons when the healers have traveled abroad.

## What Is the System's Referral Network?

Word-of-mouth testimony by satisfied patients is the only referral system used. Some travel agencies have promoted tours that include visits to the local healing chapels and practitioners. These "healing tours" were most popular in the early 1970s. Several individuals are still currently promoting legitimate healing tours to the Philippines. These organizations initially drew on the attention of some fraudulent practitioners. The tours also created a network of graft paid to taxi drivers and others who brought tourists to "fake" practitioners (Wright & Wright, 1974, p. 73). This practice has diminished, as has the popularity of Westerners seeking this alternative treatment in the Philippines.

## Are There Specialist Practitioners?

All espiritistas are specialists in that they have developed a gift for trance mediumship. Magnetic healers and psychic surgeons are the two main types of specialist practitioners among the Filipino espiritistas. The espiritistas may have specific talents that make use of their personal styles of healing. Not all healers perform psychic surgery. Many espiritistas utilize other indigenous methods, such as herbal remedies, *hilot* massage (native to the Philippines), incantations or prayer, along with other ancient traditional Asian healing modalities, such as the diagnostic techniques of pulse taking, Ayurvedic medicine, and cupping.

Orbito's Healers' Circle, an international group of healers, included a vast array of specialists. Orbito himself practiced distance healing, magnetic healing, and psychic surgery. Westerner Harvey Martin, a minister of the Healers' Circle who had also engaged in mediumship training, was a chiropractor who performed chiropractic manipulations on the psychic surgeons and their relatives in the early 1980s.

## What Kinds of Specialists Are There?

Espiritistas in the Philippines have different gifts or specializations, the ability to perform various forms of healings such as distance healing, materialization, spiritual injections, or distance cutting. For example, Alex Orbito told patients who were waiting in line to be treated by him, in Hawaii, that they should write their contact information on a piece of paper, along with the health problems they suffered from, so that he could perform "distance healing" on them. He would pray for them and heal them from a distance (Martin, 1998). Some of the more powerful healers claim to incorporate teleportation or materialization in their healing methods (as described in the Western literature review). The best known specialists were Juan Blanche, for his distance cutting; Jose Mercado, for his spiritual injections; and Josephina Sison, who was able to manipulate soft objects (cotton, cloth), apparently inserting them into the patient's body and removing them from another area, in order to effect cleansing and healing.

Espiritistas may use other methods of alleged psychic healing as well. Espiritistas may bless medicines, oil, or water for future medicinal use. McDowall (1998) reports:

> He said he would make medicine water. Water was poured from a sealed, commercial, two-liter bottle, Jun Labo placed a Bible on top of the glass and prayed to bring the prayer session to a close. He then took the Bible off the top of the glasses and we saw the water had become red. All of us were invited to sip this colored water to help in healing our diseases and building our spirituality. (p. 136)

## What Are the Usual Therapeutic Practice Sites?

In the province of Pangnasian, a rural area, the practice sites are located in remote areas. However, in Baguio City, Manila, and other more urban areas, the chapels are located in more accessible neighborhood locations. Practitioners have healing chapels that are usually assembled in a simple room either in or adjacent to their own home. The room may have a cot or several cots for the patients to use during treatment. There is generally a shrine area, with various photographs, religious icons, and candles. Water and oils, which are blessed during worship services, are placed on the shrine, along with candles, holy images, such as the image of Santo Ninio, and other objects of special importance to the healer.

## What Are the System's Internal and External Legitimization and Oversight Structures?

Generally, traditional or folk medicine, in existence since ancient times, has not been validated by scientific research. With the advent of scientific experimentation and instrumentation, these forms of healing, especially in Western countries, have been ridiculed and opposed by most established medical practitioners. Even in Asia, the home of traditional healing practices in this modern age, "Folk healing is often looked upon with suspicion by the scientific community"(Licauco, 1999 p. 139).

There is very little external oversight of the alleged healing practices of espiritistas and other indigenous healers in the Philippines. The Union of Espiritistas of the Philippines endorses its own healers. The espiritistas have attended mediumship trainings and seminars where they have been assisted in developing their spiritual gifts and skill of mediumship. The original group of healers had a banner in front of their home or chapel bearing the name of The Union of Espiritistas of the Philippines. They are more recently provided a written credential from that organization for attending the mediumship training.

## What Therapeutic Measures Are Undertaken at Home or Elsewhere, on One's Own or With the Aid of Family Members?

Patients are encouraged to seek union with God and to continue their spiritual development, through prayer and worship, in whatever religion to which they may belong. In the Philippines, the general population is primarily Catholic, with some Protestant congregations; individuals will also worship and pray according to their traditional means. The Spiritist church members are likely to participate in mediumship training as a part of their prayer and worship. Patients may pray, receive distance healing, or drink blessed water. Family members may rub blessed oil on the patient and assist in other nurturing behaviors or rituals.

## How Are Practitioners Compensated?

Practitioners are compensated through donations from their patients. Sometimes the espiritista will specify the amount of compensation, although it is still referred to as a donation. The espiritistas generally receive modest, even meager compensation from local Filipinos. The donations are generally based on what one can afford. Therefore, some wealthy and very grateful Filipinos or Westerners may bestow very expensive gifts or large sums of cash. There are many accounts of espiritistas receiving Rolex watches or cars as payment for their services. It is reported by Licauco and others that Emilio Laporga received his large house and clinic from a grateful patient. When I asked Laporga (personal communication, May 23, 2001) how much he charged for an operation, he said "by donation" while practicing in the Philippines. He reported that when he traveled to foreign countries, he charged flat rates for his treatments to cover traveling expenses.

## How Does the System Interact With Other CAM Systems?

The Philippines is a country that embraces a variety of Asian and southeastAsian indigenous healing systems, including acupuncture and Ayurvedic medicine, which Westerners consider alternative. The Filipino espiritistas do not promote the avoidance of other healing systems. Espiritistas may recommend herbal remedies or other "alternative" methods of treatment. Patients may be referred to other indigenous practitioners. On occasion, espiritistas have referred patients to biomedical practitioners.

## Specific Activities and Materia Medica

## What Do Practitioners Do?

The practitioners perform so-called magnetic healing through the laying on of hands and engage in spirit-directed psychic surgeries while in trance states. After going into trance, the espiritistas act as mediums for the Holy Spirit. The Holy Spirit, working through the medium, diagnoses and treats illnesses with the techniques of magnetic healing, minor surgeries, spirit-directed psychic surgery, and sleight-of-hand psychic surgeries.

Several espiritistas admitted to Martin (1998), who had become a minister of the Healers' Circle, that sometimes espiritistas use therapeutic sleight-of-hand in their practice of psychic surgery. They were comfortable in what they were doing, since the practice of therapeutic sleight-of-hand is based on ancient Filipino healing practices. The espiritistas do not perceive this as an unethical practice. Like shamans, they base the validity of their choice of healing methods on positive outcomes.

## What Is the Specific Materia Medica?

Christian symbolism of blessed oils, candles, religious images, and icons represents the healing energy of a Christian God and reinforces the faith and belief of patients in the healer and the healing process. The espiritistas are acknowledged by reputation within the local community and are recognized by their altars, shrines, and banners. The espiritistas' altars may include many religious pictures, symbols, and candles that are lit during the healing transactions. There are often sets of three candles representing the Holy Trinity of God the Father, God the Son, and God the Holy Spirit. People bring water and oil to the shrines to be blessed by the espiritistas prior to the healing transactions.

The espiritistas bless their medicines and will even bless Western pharmaceuticals prior to patients ingesting them. The espiritista often dips his or her fingers in one or more blessed oils and then draws a cross on the patient's forehead or back before diagnosing and treating. Some espiritistas claim that spirit guides assist them in gathering information and diagnosing while they are touching the patients. A psychic surgeon's main set of tools are his bare hands. Some specific materials used at the healer's location are a cot or table prepared for the patient with a sheet or blanket, blessed oil and water, sometimes cotton balls, towels, or other medical supplies.

## What Are the Classes and Purposes of Interventions?

Magnetic healing, minor surgeries, spirit-directed psychic surgery, and sleight-of-hand psychic surgeries are all classes of interventions provided by the Filipino espiritistas. The espiritistas may also utilize techniques of spirit-directed medicine by performing distance healing, blessing water or other medicines, spiritual injections, the ancient art of cupping, and more.

The stated purpose of magnetic healing and psychic surgery are to restore both physical and spiritual balance. Therapeutic actions include the removing of so-called negative energies and restoring healthy energies, removing or dissolving diseased tissues, and restoring tissues to a healthy state. Spiritual injections, such as performed by Mercado, are for the maintenance of health. Other indigenous practitioners provide a wide range of alternative treatments. For the Filipino espiritistas, all illnesses exist in the spiritual realm as well as the physical realm; treatment is provided for both simultaneously.

# Responsibilities

## What Are the Responsibilities of Practitioners?

The Filipino espiritistas embrace Christian beliefs and a broad worldview in their spiritual practices. The espiritistas are responsible to pray, worship God diligently, to receive the training, and develop their skills of mediumship to allow the Holy Spirit to heal through them unobstructed (the state of *nabuksan*).

While the Catholics attribute healing to an act of God, most westerners with an allopathic frame of reference erroneously perceive the psychic surgeon to be totally responsible for the healing process. Psychic surgeons, however, believe that it is the power of the Holy Spirit working through them that actually performs the operations. It is not their work, but the work of the Spirit.

Espiritistas are expected to diligently worship God, to maintain their spiritual development, and to continue to serve others with their healing gifts. However, contrary to these notions, many espiritistas act as trickster character types (see Discussion section). According to Hansen (2001), controversies and dichotomies created by the "trickster" may increase personal power, charisma, and authority in many different cultures worldwide.

## What Are the Responsibilities of Patients or Clients?

There are many deliberate ritual acts performed during the course of treatment. The patient's role is mostly passive during the healing session, although the person may be asked to participate in some type of ritual over the course of several days. Patients may drink holy water or rub oil on themselves. They may be required to ingest written "prescriptions" (spirit writing) by chewing up the paper or drinking the water from containers that contain the written prescription. Patients may be told to ask for forgiveness for their sins and to attend to their spiritual development. As Alex Orbito explained to Martin (1998),

> When I give spiritual healing to your body, as long as you are doing good, the cure will be effective. But if you are doing bad, the spiritual healing will disappear and the influence of the negative will return. That is why you must continue your spiritual development. (pp. 16-17)

Clients may be instructed to go and sin no more and to continue their spiritual development. Sin is seen as a frequent cause of illness, hence, for many patients, repentance will represent a lifestyle change.

Patients are responsible for their daily thoughts, words, and deeds, and for striving to live in harmony with God.

> Many people actually receive their healing but, most often, let it slip through their fingers. New converts should feed on the Word of God. They should be filled with the Spirit; they should make prayer a daily habit. Their lives then become filled with faith and with God. There is no room for Satan to return. (Agpaoa, as cited in Martin 2002b, pp. 40-41)

Spiritual development is the responsibility of the individual, although the espiritista, during the healing processes, may inspire the continuation of their spiritual growth through prayer and worship. Some espiritistas emphasize this aspect of the healing process and some do not.

## What Are the Responsibilities of Family or Community Members?

Family and community members can participate in worship and spiritual growth along with the patient.

> One of the most common mistakes made by those who oppose the ministry of divine healing is that they utterly fail to realize that divine healing is governed not by magic, but by definite laws. Healing is by faith, and that faith is supplied by three sources: the one who prays for the sick, those who have brought the person, and the patient himself. Some faith is required of each one of the parties involved. (Agpaoa, as cited in Martin 2002b, p. 40)

Families in the Philippines are strongly united. Even distant family members (e.g., cousins, uncles, aunts) may be obligated to provide money for the cost of treatment or transportation for the patients. Otherwise these strong family ties may have little effect on the patients and healers.

## Are There Consensual Ethical Norms?

When people go to an espiritista for healing, they are consenting to be treated with great respect by the practitioner. There are no specific consensual ethical norms generally. The espiritistas are rarely specific in regards to the mechanisms of their interventions, unlike in the West, where informed consent exists as an ethical standard and the practitioner is required to provide information regarding risks, side effects, and so on. For example, patients are not told when the application of sleight-of-hand psychic surgery will be used. This information would perhaps negate the placebo effect inherent in the treatment.

Some espiritistas claim the patients do not need to have faith, although the espiritistas themselves do need to experience faith in powers of nabuksan. Espiritistas say the patient's religion is not a concern. It is best if one believes in God, in whatever manner God is perceived by the individual. There is also the implicit assumption that patients will trust the practitioner and the process.

## Scope

## How Extensive, Varied, or Specialized Are the System's Applications?

The applications of this healing system are varied and specialized. The practice of mediumship, psychic surgery, distance cutting, spiritual injections, and the expulsion of evil spirits are all fairly unique to this system and are rarely found in other cultures in this specific constellation. The practitioners do not specialize in particular physical ailments; rather, they specialize in their own particular form of healing intervention (e.g., minor surgery, spirit directed psychic surgery, sleight-of- hand psychic surgery). The espiritistas treat nearly all forms of illness and all types, ages, and ethnic groups of people. Some practitioners seem more adept at going "deeper" into the physical body, while others generally operate on tumors and cists that are close to the body's surface, just under the skin.

## Analysis of Benefits and Barriers

## What Are the Risks and Costs of the System From the Insider's Perspective?

Proponents of the Western biomedical model claim there is a great risk of utilizing this system of faith healing, warning that psychic surgery is sought out by those who refuse the use of standard medical practices. According to Nolen (1974), patients are taking a great risk by neglecting medical treatment that may be more effective in curing certain ailments. He also stated that it may be a risk for foreigners to travel to the Philippines, as the climate is extreme and the trip can be long and stressful, presenting a hardship for seriously ill people.

From the insider's perspective, the expenses of practitioners and/or the cost to patients utilizing this system of healing are minimal. A few pesos are an acceptable amount for local Filipinos to pay for services of espiritistas. Donations for the healer's services are individually determined, based on patient satisfaction and ability to pay.

The practitioners I observed did not especially emphasize sin or sinful behavior as the cause of ailments. But if a practitioner over emphasizes sinful behavior as the cause of the patient's ailments, this might produce guilt reactions that would be counterproductive. Guilt could result in unsuccessful interventions.

## Accommodation and Views of Suffering and Death

## How Does the System View Suffering and Death?

The espiritistas hold a conservative Christian notion about suffering. God will allow suffering so that lessons of compassion or humility can be learned. However, unlike most Christians, the espiritistas believe in reincarnation. They accept the existence of a spiritual realm, and they believe that human spirits exist intact and can communicate from that realm with the physical world. They perceive death simply as a transition, one stage in a spiritual continuum. One can minimize suffering and prepare for death through spiritual growth. "You live after death. We believe in that.

We have proof of it through our spirit mediums (espiritistas). They [the spirits, speaking through mediums] give us messages. We are in constant touch with the other world" (Tolentino, cited in Sherman, 1966, p. 78).

## Comparison and Interaction With Dominant System
## What Does the System Provide for Healing and for Coping With Illness That the Dominant System Does Not Provide?

Espiritistas provide healing mostly in the spiritual realm, which then leads to healing of the physical body, whereas Western biomedicine addresses only physical illness, symptom alleviation, and minor preventatives, leaving spiritual concerns to others. It is also reported that the espiritistas are quite successful with certain ailments with which allopathic medicine is less successful (Licauco, 1999). The espiritistas encourage worship of God and spiritual growth. They also provide treatment for malign human agency or witchcraft, which Western biomedical doctors do not.

Folk and faith healing in the Philippines is the dominant system of healing-its history is long and its roots deep. Additionally, there is widespread economic disadvantage in this county, which prevents access to pharmaceutical medicine. Typically, there is minimal interaction with the allopathic practitioners by the middle and lower classes, although there are a few exceptions. The espiritistas provide a vehicle for belief in God and a way to find a spiritual path. They promote spiritual growth as a means to wellness.

This system of healing provides a spiritually oriented healing dynamic focusing on faith, belief in God, and the healing power of the Holy Spirit. The dominant system of healing does not recognize spiritual components of illness and healing, and it neglects the treatment of any aspects of illness that arise from sources other than those that can be explained from a biomedical perspective. Generally, medical interventions consist of pharmaceuticals or invasive surgery. Filipino faith healing and psychic surgery provide a strong spiritual component to health, healing, and illness that is not present in the practice of Western medicine. The patients who utilize this system are given both spiritual and physical treatment.

## How Does This System View Interaction With the Dominant System?

In rural areas of the Philippines, folk healing is the dominant system of healing, which is not the norm for most modern nations. There is little interaction between the Filipino espiritistas and the Western practitioners of biomedicine, both in the Philippines and abroad. It is alleged that sometimes espiritistas will refer patients to medical doctors. For example, Nolen (1974) reported that Terte and Agpaoa had referred patients to allopathic practitioners. Agpaoa's alleged referral was made after his patient had returned to the United States and was still suffering from symptoms. Espiritistas do not report being opposed to networking with allopathic practitioners, and, occasionally, they will refer someone for allopathic medicine.

Juan Labo (cited in McDowall, 1998) commented on the interaction between Western medicine and psychic surgery. He stated, "There should be closer cooperation between western medicine and psychic healing" (p. 181). Labo was frequently in conflict with the Philippine Medical Association, because patients with seemingly incurable conditions would be kept in hospitals for months before being released with no further options. After being released to their homes, many would go to

Labo and allegedly were cured. The medical association took credit for their cures and the medicines they had used. Labo reports he did not blame the doctors' attitudes as much as their training. He maintains that there should be a way to facilitate the collaboration of Western medicine and folk healing. The World Health Organization (WHO) has for years been promoting the integration of traditional medicine into mainstream health care.

> A WHO meeting on the promotion and development of Traditional medicine was held in Geneva from 28 November to 2 December 1977. The aim of the meeting was therefore to assemble expert representatives of the major systems of traditional medicine to work together and suggest a plan of action to promote and develop the various aspects of traditional medicine. (World Health Organization, 1977, p. 7)

"Traditional medicine (TRM) in Pacific islands is an old, ancestral health system which has remained practically unchanged for many centuries. Practitioners of TRM are mainly herbalists, bone-setters, masseuses, and faith healers" (World Health Organization, 2002, p. 9). In 1990, a team of six Filipino doctors performed research into the practices of the local *manghihilots* (bone setters) to evaluate their roles in the community and to explore the possibility of integrating the manghihilots into the health care system. The team found the diagnostics and methods of treatment by the manghihilots as adequate and appropriate for primary health care in the community. However, the Philippine Medical Association is nowhere near accepting spiritists whose practice borders on the paranormal into their health care system.

In urban areas of the Philippines, Western medicine is firmly rooted and, after generations of Western modernization, members of the Philippine Medical Association warned clinics they would lose their licenses if they continued to work with the indigenous folk or faith healers. WHO's efforts to combine allopathic medicine with indigenous healing practices has "a long way to go" (Licauco, 1992,

p. 141). WHO has provided support to the Philippines "to develop plans for traditional medicine programs at the national level and a training package for traditional healers, with a simple message on basic principles of preventing disease and promoting health" (World Health Organization, 2000, p. 2). In spite of this support, there is an extremely minimal amount of interaction between the Filipino espiritistas and Western biomedicine.

There have been very few clinical trials or other forms of research on the Filipino espiritistas. Of all the nations in the world, Brazil seems to be one country where both the practice of Kardec-influenced spiritism and psychical research flourish within mainstream society (H. Martin, personal communication, November 18, 2002). A recent article written by Aliso Viejo (2000) regarding clinical trials, "Trance Surgery in Brazil," was published in *Alternative Therapies in Health and Medicine*. "An in-depth study of safety and clinical efficacy of these extreme practices [psychic surgery] remains to be performed.

Greenfield surveyed 32 patients of Mauricio Magalhaes," whose methods of mediumship supposedly incorporate the spirit of Dr. Adolph Fritz (cited in Viejo, 2000, p. 5). Dr. Fritz was one of the discarnate spirit entities Arigo and others claimed to be possessed by during their alleged "possession states" and healing practices (Fuller, 1974, p. 54). These Brazilian practitioners perform Kardec influenced spiritism and psychic surgery similar to the Filipino espiritistas.

# VII. MEDIUMSHIP AND PSYCHIC SURGERY AS INDIGENOUS HEALING PHENOMENA

## Other Theoretical Perspectives

Many of the espiritistas have been identified as mediums who claim to channel bisa, or the power of the Holy Spirit. The psychic surgeons can be placed with the Kardec-influenced spiritists, who are similar to the trance mediums who practice psychic surgery in Brazil. Most of the lesser known Filipino espiritistas are referred to as tambalans or mananambal and practice a more traditional Filipino form of trance healing, although they are similarly Christian and refer to the source of their healing power as that of the Holy Spirit.

Michael Winkelman's (1992) schema is employed to place the espiritistas in the context of other indigenous healers and the diverse practices of Filipino folk and faith healing. To further define this system of healing, this research model and several suppositions, including Hansen's (2001) trickster character type and an explanation of shamanic trickery according to Walsh (1990), will frame the context from which the practice of psychic surgery evolved.

## Winkelman's Schema

Winkelman (1984) performed a meta-analysis of anthropological and sociological studies and magico-religious phenomena, and he has published numerous writings on the topic of shamanism. He later revised his original schema and published his theories in *Shamans, Priests and*

*Witches: A Cross-Cultural Study of Magico-Religious Practitioners* (1992). His classification system for categorizing *shamanistic* practitioners is a result of correlations made between the social complexity of a community and its culturally defined healing practices. Winkelman contends that the healers' duties depend on various types of altered states of consciousness (ASC). The schema of magico-religious practices is used here to classify the espiritistas within the context of other indigenous Filipino healers.

Winkelman's (1992) unique classification system includes descriptions of these practices of ASC and how they correlate with social complexity and political integration. Winkelman begins his categorical system with the Shaman, practicing in the simplest cultures. He proceeds to add components of social complexity and corresponding healer types: shaman/healer, healer, medium, priest, and malevolent practitioner (sorcerer/ witch). All of Winkelman's classifications exist in the Philippines; four of these types of healers are prevalent in this country with its broad spectrum of niche cultures, from indigenous to modern. Difficult traveling conditions and the unique geography of this 7,000-island archipelago account for the small diverse cultural niches and the variety of healing practices in the Philippines.

According to Winkelman (1992), a magico-religious practitioner labeled a shaman can be found in the most simple classless societies throughout the world. "Shamans were found only in societies with no formal classes or in semi-nomadic hunting and gathering (or fishing) societies lacking agriculture and without administrative political organization beyond the local community" (Winkelman, 1984, pp. 10-11).

Rebecca Tiston (1983) claims shamanism is still practiced in the more rural isolated areas of the Philippines, such as in Northern Leyte.

> The Tambalan is conceived to have possessed power from higher spirits in that he has power over other spirits. He journeys to the sky to meet the heavenly beings face to face in order to present an offering for and in behalf of his patients. He goes elsewhere in the

universe in search of the soul of the sick believed to be wandering around decoyed by the human spirits of departed ancestors; and finally goes to the heavens of the land of the spirits in order to learn deeper truths by conversing with them." (p. 9)

In societies similar to those of the Philippines that developed agriculture and sedentary lifestyles, the shaman becomes transformed into the more specialized role of shaman healer. The primary activities of the shaman healer are divination and healing; they also provide protection against spirits or malevolent magical practitioners. Winkelman contends that the healers, the third member of the Shaman Complex, are strongly predicted by the presence of political integration beyond the local level. This applies to the Filipino espiritistas who were influenced by the colonization of the Philippine islands by Spain 400 years ago. In societies with hierarchical political systems, the shaman healers undergo further transformation into the healer role, largely omitting trance states.

Winkelman (1992) promotes that healer types are most likely to be found in societies that rely upon agriculture for their primary source of food (p.12).

> Statistics of 1990 reveal 47% of the Filipinos people are employed in agriculture, fishery and forestry, followed by 17.5% who are in the services, community, social and personal. Wholesale and retail trade make up 13.1%, while manufacturing is 10.3%. (Panopio, Cordero-MacDonald, & Raymundo, 1994, p. 238)

The diverse peoples of the Philippines are relying more on industrialization. With increased urbanization and exposure to international influences, Filipinos form a complex society that is rapidly becoming Westernized. However, the islands currently remain rich with numerous indigenous practitioners who continue to perform magic-religious healing. Their healing systems, based on ancient *shamanic* modes, have been diluted by the cultural demands of Westernization and the influence of the Catholic Church. The more complex a society, the more likely it is to have representatives fitting Winkelman's schema in its entirety.

The Philippine islands make up the only Asian country where the majority of the people are of the Christian faith. The Philippine people have also been greatly influenced by modern American culture, both socially and politically, since they were once a territory of the United States. The result of this interesting blend of indigenous, Asian, European, and American cultures has been a great diversity in worldview among the country's native and immigrant peoples. The espiritistas, however, owe their cultural roots to the islands' indigenous shamanic cultures.

The Christian-influenced Filipino espiritistas act as mediums, claiming to heal with the power of the Holy Spirit. Their practices are related to the shamanic realm in regard to their voluntary control of shifts of consciousness. The Kardec-influenced espiritistas and many of the other tambalans are a good fit for Winkelman's category of mediums. Espiritistas establish practices that include folk, religious, and spiritual knowledge specific to illness and healing. The espiritistas utilize their individual talents for altering their states of consciousness, and they engage in formal training from other espiritistas in the skill of channeling the Holy Spirit. It is believed that mediums call spiritual entities into their bodies. "The term medium is selected because they engage in some form of possession alternate state of consciousness (ASC), during which spirits are believed to take over the medium's body and operate through it" (Winkelman, 1992, p. 59).

Ruth-Inge Heinze (1997), following her extensive experience in Southeast Asia studying trance mediums, describes shamans as employing alternate states of consciousness during consultations, divinations, and healing. Heinze (1991) states, "It is important to mention that, especially in Asia, shamans also act as spirit mediums" (p. 10). They respond to specific needs in their community, which are otherwise not fulfilled, and act as mediators between the sacred and the secular, utilizing different states of consciousness. Mediums do not generally use magical techniques, but instead rely upon their ASC relationships with spirits and propitiation as a means of manipulating the supernatural (Heinze, 1997).

In the Philippines, it is the influence of political integration and the presence of the Catholic Church within Philippine society that most influence shamanic practices. The healers, priests, malevolent practitioners, and mediums exist in Philippine society where the Catholic Church is significantly established. However, the mediums have been pushed to the fringes of society and back into the rural areas, where they originally existed during early Spanish colonization.

The priest category of magico-religious healing arises in societies with increased political stratification, affected by the growth of commerce and industrialization. In the Philippines the influence of the Catholic Church has also been instrumental in the socio-political hierarchy. Some Catholic Filipinos utilize services from healers, as well as from priests of the Catholic Church or charismatic ministers of Protestant Christian churches. "Some Filipino priests practice exorcism, prayer healing, and some magico-religious practices" (D. Taubold, personal communication, November 10, 2002).

Other prominent roles of magico-religious practitioners in the Philippines are the malevolent practitioners, the witches and sorcerers. According to Winkelman (1992) these practices originated in the shamanic type practitioner but acquired their unique characteristics as a result of their persecution by the healers and priests. Malevolent practitioners are generally thought to have low social or economic status and can be either male or female in most societies. Malevolent practitioners frequently acquire their role through social labeling, rather than seeking such on the part of the individual. 'The data suggest that there is continuity between those malevolent practitioners acting deliberately and those engaged in unconscious psychic acts, with the latter found in societies with higher levels of political integration" (Winkelman, 1984, p. 5). The Philippines, being a complex society, include all of Winkelman's classified practitioners. Hansen (2001) elaborates on Winkelman's model in relation to priests and mediums and describes his contentions about the trickster character type.

## Hansen's Trickster Character Type

Hansen (2001) was employed in parapsychological laboratories for 8 years (3 years at Rhine Research Center and 5 years at Princeton) and is a member of the Brotherhood of Magicians. He mentions the Filipino psychic surgeons in his book *The Trickster and the Paranormal*. He elaborates on shamans and mediums and their frequent use of both psi and magic. Hansen also elaborates on the dynamics proposed by Winkelman. "In ancient times priests became differentiated from magicians, as injunctions were placed against the use of magic" (p. 105). The Filipino espiritistas experienced this occurrence with the coming of the Catholic priests.

According to Hansen (2001), Winkelman's schema clearly identifies the important relationships between societal structure and the status of purported psi practitioners. In the Philippines, the high status and visibility of Catholic priests and medical doctors exemplify this, as well as the societal invisibility of mediums prior to their popular exposure to the West in the early 1960s. "Supernatural powers have been recognized for thousands of years" (p. 101).

Yet, as societies become complex, the practitioners who attempt to delve into supernatural practices are shunted to the margins; they are denigrated as crazy, epileptic, or deviant, just as the psychic surgeons in the Philippines have been. This labeling promoted by established science, Western biomedicine, and the Catholic Church helped preserve the established hierarchy of medical practitioners, politicians, and organized religion. Purported direct contact with psi and the paranormal is antistructural, and, in Philippine society, it is found on the fringe of society. The institutions of science and biomedicine are elite, exclusive, and hierarchical in structure (p. 101).

These dynamics are consistent with the Filipino espiritistas who claim to practice the art of mediumship, psi healing, and the use of therapeutic sleight-of-hand. The Catholic Church and medical practitioners of the allopathic model have persecuted them. Persecution from the priests and the medical professionals pushed the espiritistas to the fringes of their society. However, the popularity of these practices in the 1960s and through the 1970s brought much needed foreign income to the Philippine Islands, which resulted in some tolerance from the political leaders at that time. For example, Ferdinand Marcos, the former president of the Philippines, was treated by espiritistas and promoted the utilization of their practices.

Of all the practitioners considered here, shamans and mediums make the most use of altered states of consciousness; they directly and intentionally engage purported paranormal powers. Based upon the findings of parapsychology, it can be expected that shamans and mediums make the most use of psi. They also have the greatest number of trickster characteristics and are particularly associated with deception. (Hansen, 2001, p. 101)

Hansen (2001) contends that the Filipino espiritistas are good examples of the trickster character type. He borrows from a cross disciplinary approach to describe the character type he refers to as the *trickster*. According to Hansen, "The trickster is a character type found in mythology, folklore, and literature the world over" (p. 28). Hansen's approach is eclectic; he draws from mythology, folklore, history, parapsychology, anthropology, psychology, religion, and psychiatry. He contends that "Boundaries must be blurred for the trickster to be seen" (p. 29).

> Tricksters have a number of common characteristics, and some of their most salient qualities are disruption, unrestrained sexuality, disorder, and nonconformity to the establishment... The trickster unifies major, but seemingly unrelated themes surrounding the paranormal. For instance, the paranormal is frequently connected with deception, and deceit is second nature to the trickster. (pp. 28-36)

The Filipino espiritistas practice their unique blend of spiritism and healing outside the mainstream medical and religious communities. Many of the psychical researchers, reporters, and laypersons, trickster types in their own right, also practice outside the mainstream scientific and academic communities, as do the healers they investigate. Hansen's cross-disciplinary approach is consistent with this project's methodology, utilizing widely varied sources. Written accounts come from the varied disciplines of history, psychology, psychical research, anthropology, religion, and both allopathic and complementary and alternative forms of medicine.

A good example of the trickster figure is Ormond McGill, who was one of the first psychical investigators to travel to the Philippines to observe psychic surgery. Hansen (2001) elaborates on the career of McGill as a trickster type.

> He authored *The Encyclopedia of Stage Hypnotism* (1947) a manual used by numerous stage performers. He was also involved in debates on psychic phenomena. McGill not only held a positive view on the reality of psi, but he even gave advice on how to fake them, in the 1940s. In the 1970s he published several popular books describing his travels and encounters with supernatural phenomena. (p. 141)

McGill filmed the espiritista Eleuterio Terte in 1958, and Harold Sherman, a psychical researcher, filmed Tony Agpaoa in 1965. Agpaoa was the most prominent of the Philippine healers in the early 1970s. He was the psychic surgeon who best exemplified the trickster character type. Agpaoa was an independent practitioner who did not belong to the Union of Espiritistas of the Philippines and did not exhibit the Christian Spiritists' humility, as did the other healers at this time.

Agpaoa was a businessman who had been charging money for his services, and he was accused of fraud on numerous occasions. Agpaoa, a rural commoner whose gift for healing had only been appreciated by local Filipinos, suddenly became an international sensation, and the attention he received enhanced his many trickster characteristics.

Brother David Oligani [refers to Tony] as a healer who refuses even donations to his church and shed genuine tears when he contemplated brother Tony. All he could say was, I do not understand brother Tony. In the eyes of this practicing man of God, Tony Agpaoa has committed sacrilege. (Valentine, 1973, pp. 94-95)

Regarding Tony Agpaoa, Valentine (1973) states, "For every story that alleges fraud, I can dig up two that claim he's a miracle worker" (p. 31). The womanizing, gambling, and allegations of fraud seemed to add to the popularity of the personality of Tony Agpaoa, the psychic surgeon trickster of the Philippines. Jun Labo, another psychic surgeon, previously the Mayor of Baguio City, and a prominent businessman, was married several times and was a controversial figure who also became somewhat of a trickster character type.

Many of the Filipino espiritistas fit Hansen's trickster character type. Hansen (2001) further promotes the idea that, "Marginality and anti-structure are associated with attempts to explicitly engage psi" (p. 424). Methodologies for investigating psi practices often begin with defining the intervention. What exactly is the healer doing? One must define the healing intervention before further research can occur. It is difficult to determine what a trickster is doing. It is in their interest to remain mysterious, and their practices remain difficult to comprehend. The Filipino espiritistas do not usually admit to the use of therapeutic sleight-of-hand. According to Krippner (1976), Martin (1998), and others, the Filipino espiritistas perform minor surgical procedures and both spirit-directed psychic surgery and sleight-of-hand psychic surgery. Sleight-of-hand, which is a technique of Hansen's trickster character type, can also be viewed as shamanic trickery.

## Walsh and Shamanic Trickery

In *The Spirit of Shamanism,* Roger Walsh, M.D., Ph. D., a professor of psychiatry, philosophy, and anthropology at the University of California at Irvine, elaborates on the traditional shaman's use of therapeutic sleight-of-hand. According to Walsh (1990), it is clear that shamans may engage in all manners of trickery. Shamanic trickery is performed not purely for the shaman's benefit but for the benefit of the patient. Shamanism and shamanic practices are valuable and effective in their own right. It would be difficult to determine if shamans use more trickery than other healers and professionals. Walsh contends it is clear that, while shamans may indulge in trickery, shamanism cannot be dismissed as only trickery. The healing potential of psychic surgery, which, at times, may include the practice of some "trickery" or therapeutic sleight of-hand, is of appropriate interest to humanistic psychologists, due to its effects on the human condition, the healing potential that incorporates faith and belief, as well as other aspects of human consciousness in the processes of illness and healing (pp. 104-109).

According to Walsh (1990), trickery is far more than an act of fraud. Some shamans are most definitely tricksters, but this in no way indicates that all shamans are only tricksters. It is, therefore, possible that shamans may use some oftheirtricks quite consciously to increase their therapeutic impact. The Filipino espiritistas increase their therapeutic impact and often facilitate cathartic experiences for their patients with the use of psychic surgery (p. 104).

# VIII. DISCUSSION

This study proposed the question: Does fit the descriptive parameters for complementary and alternative medicine? This delimitation permitted focus on the system itself, not the issues of the system's effectiveness, its utilization of anomalous mechanisms, or its similarities to other folk healing systems. A large body of archival data has been applied to the CAM parameters that produced a description of the Filipino espirtistas' system of healing. After reviewing the application of the archival data to the CAM parameters, the determination was made that the Filipino espiritistas' system of healing is a good fit with the CAM parameters for a complementary or alternative healing system.

Essential elements and common factors in healing are revealed in the espiritistas' beliefs and practices. The description of a system of healing must be provided as a starting point for further research, especially of esoteric systems that utilize mind-body medicine and are on the margin of paranormal. A discussion of how the Filipino espiritistas fit with the other systems of healing models by Kleinman, Frank and Frank, and Torrey will be followed by the current limitations presented by Brody and Brody (2000), presenting other issues regarding the Filipino espiritistas' system of healing and the role of human consciousness in illness and healing experiences.

## Martin: The Secret Teachings of the Espiritistas

Martin (1998) reported his experience of coming to an understanding of the espiritistas' use of sleight-of-hand psychic surgery. Reverend Benjamin Pajarillo explained to Martin, a minister of the

Healers' Circle, that he had observed some psychic surgeons who were very skilled at constructing performances of therapeutic sleight-of-hand. Martin became concerned about who were "real" healers and who were not. Martin questioned Pajarillo, "How could anyone possibly determine who the real healers were if sleight-of hand could produce healing miracles?" Pajarillo replied that "a real healer is one who restores health" (p. 158).

> Sleight of hand psychic surgery was not merely a 'fake' simulation of 'genuine' psychic surgery that the healer used when his powers waned. Sleight of hand psychic surgery is the outcome of shamanic healing practices that have been successfully applied in the Philippines for hundreds, perhaps even thousands of years. Far from being a form of fakery, sleight of hand surgery is the natural outcome of the traditional wisdom of the ancestors of the psychic surgeons, and has been practiced in Filipino culture for centuries. (p. 162)

In another conversation, Pajarillo explained to Martin (1998) that in Western society, sleight-of-hand is the basis of parlor game entertainment and may involve pulling rabbits out of hats or other magic tricks. Yet, "if an innovative and unique use of sleight-of-hand for healing purposes that would extend the lives of incurable patients well past the expected dates of their demise, would we be foolish not to use it" (p. 160). Martin became aware of the relationship between mediumship, healing, and use of therapeutic sleight-of hand in the same way that systems of healing models presume that human consciousness plays an essential role in both the illness and healing processes of human beings (p. 160).

Martin (1998) realized that the therapeutic interventions he observed could not be limited to the simplistic dualism of being "fake" or "real." "I saw that psychological factors within the patient could render 'real' therapies useless while deriving dramatic results from 'fake' therapies" (p. 158). Martin told a number of people about his discovery, and he was shocked to find that no one believed him! None of the patients who had been successfully treated by the espiritistas and who "were 'healed' could believe that the very dramatic transformation in their health could have resulted from anything other than a genuine paranormal intervention" (pp. 158- 159). These patients' experiences can be identified by essential elements of illness and healing within the system of healing models (Appendix B).

## Kleinman's Proposal

The Filipino espiritistas claim to enter altered states of consciousness, as they become instruments of the Holy Spirit in trance. Kleinman (1988a) contends that trance and possession states are commonplace in indigenous healing systems. "In the disenchanted modern west, meditation, hypnosis, and other relaxation techniques appear to have replaced possession states as the major lay and professional forms for eliciting altered states of consciousness" (p. 123). Kleinman observed similar healing practices by the local shamans in Taiwan, which stimulated his interest in the healing dynamics of patients and healers in the context of their own cultures.

During a discussion of the placebo effect by a group of diverse scholars, Kleinman (cited in Harrington, 1997) proposed the idea that if other theories of healing were examined, much of what is regarded as the central mediators between the social and the physiological, the interpersonal and the personal, are indeed elements such as vital energy, movement, *qi*. In Chinese medicine, qi literally means movement, energy, or power. The Filipino espiritistas may utilize the same energy and refer to it as bisa or the Holy Spirit.

Kleinman contends that all forms of healing create conditions for catharsis, though some are much more effective than others at eliciting this important therapeutic process. The use of trickery (therapeutic sleight-of-hand), when framed in the context of the paranormal, can intensify the stimulation of healing dynamics to create a vital cathartic experience, alter consciousness, and change the patient's conceptualization of illness. The flamboyant and dynamic practices of some of the Filipino espiritistas certainly create catharsis, and this catharsis could account for the high percentages of positive outcomes allegedly resulting from their interventions. Where the therapeutic ethos encourages the patient's attachment to healing symbols that are neither too remote from, nor too close to, the patient's emotional experience, catharsis is more likely to occur.

Catharsis is a therapeutic process in most non-Western healing systems. "Many observers of the healing ritual have posited psychophysiological effects of autonomic nervous system arousal and psychoneuroimmunological and endocrinological activation" (Prince, cited in Kleinman, 1988a, p. 121). According to Kleinman, one of the most profound aspects of Western biomedicine that differentiates if from every other healing system in the world is its antivitalism. Nonetheless, very few serious students of healing rituals doubt that significant biological effects result from cathartic experiences. "Most psychiatrists believe that one or more of the same processes underwrite potentially powerful biological effects in psychotherapy" (Kleinman, 1988a, p. 121-123).

## Frank and Frank's Contention

In *Persuasion and Healing,* Frank and Frank (1991) traced healing systems back to a time when illness was regarded as primarily supernatural, and treatments for illnesses were magic ritual transactions that were performed to reverse the cause of the illness. Frank and Frank contend that the brain is the seat of consciousness, the control mechanism for the nervous (neurological), endocrine, and immune systems. Both attitude and expectation can affect the dynamics of illness and healing processes.

Furthermore, Frank and Frank (1991) contend that three main factors exist in the effective healing experience: (a) the instillation of hope, through "naming" or diagnosing problems within the patient's own cultural context; (b) emotional arousal and dynamic healing techniques (such as psychic surgery, which undoubtedly creates a catharsis in believing individuals); and (c) a sense of mastery and a feeling of control gained over the perceived problem, which patients can experience by living a virtuous lifestyle and making other life changes with follow-up ritual processes.

These essential elements of healing are inherent in the practices of the Filipino espiritistas. The vital and dynamic techniques utilized by the Filipino espiritistas often facilitate emotional arousal and cathartic experiences for patients that surpass the common practices of the biomedical and most other alternative healing systems.

## The Torrey Model

E. F. Torrey (1972), a clinical research psychiatrist with a background in anthropology, developed one of the earliest systems of healing models. The Torrey Model was referred to in relation to the Filipino indigenous healers by local Filipino author Rebecca Tiston (1983), in *The Tambalans of Northern Leyte.* Torrey's model is explanatory on five levels.

1. The healer's naming of the affliction within a shared worldview is a precursor to the instillation of hope.
2. The personal caring qualities of the healer facilitate recovery from an illness experience. The personal qualities of the healer (as expert, Holy Men, ortricksterfigures),combined with the expectations of the patients, promote the efficacy of alternative, mind/body medicine. Filipino indigenous healers carry an air of confidence and caring that affects their patients in a positive manner.
3. Torrey contends that expectant faith or the instillation of hope is another essential element of the healing process. Even the process of preparing to see the healer, standing in line, or waiting in a room full of others is a different experience from similar procedures in the West. In the waiting rooms, patients spoke highly of the healers and stated confidence in the treatments they were about to receive. This dynamic is consistent with

the instillation of hope or expectant faith which facilitates the healing process.
4. Torrey concluded that the materials (materia medica) used empower the patient.
5. The specific ritual acts the patient engages in empower the patient.

The chapels or altars of the Filipino healers are filled with symbols of the Christian faith-pictures of Christ with light surrounding his head; images of the healing Saint, Santo Ninio; and candles and oils are the most common artifacts. The healing rituals working in concert with these special materials, which are familiar to the patient, promote positive expectations, and the patient's faith and belief promote healing. Most Westerners would refer to this faith healing as a placebo effect. Brody and Brody (2000) more accurately describe the process as a placebo response. They perceive that aspects of meaning (faith and belief) activate the "inner pharmacy" (p. 140).

According to the proponents of systems of healing models, the patients' faith and belief, combined with patients' expectations of the indigenous healers, promote their inner healing processes. This process is consistent with Brody and Brody and their concept of an inner pharmacy. Martin's contention that the psychic surgeon's sleight-of-hand promotes a placebo effect is supportive of the systems of healing models, regarding the role of consciousness in both illness and healing responses. The essential elements of the systems of healing approach, the healing principles, and the common factors in healing (Appendix B) can be identified in the Filipino espiritistas' system of healing, including the practice of psychic surgery. The experience of psychic surgery, for example, may result in a catharsis or a placebo response that can stimulate the inner pharmacy and increase the body's own natural healing abilities.

# IX. LIMITATIONS AND ISSUES

Although the healing mechanisms used by the espiritistas are difficult to determine according to empirical science, Walsh (1990) contends that "we can assess the possibility of psi-induced healing in shamanism in several ways" (p. 195). The claims of psychic abilities in religious and other esoteric healing traditions, anecdotal reports, and laboratory studies of psi in shamans are all open for examination. Walsh promotes further research in psi healing. "We can examine similarities between shamanic healing rituals and those conditions reported to maximize psi" (p.195).

The technology does not yet exist to verify the mechanisms and efficacy of the techniques and procedures utilized by the Filipino espiritistas from the esoteric perspective, such as the reported intervention of the Holy Spirit or the use of psi in paranormal healing. Current technologies cannot demonstrate psi beyond the possibility of the effects of secondary-interaction effects (Stelter, 1976). Heinze (1997) contends:

> Without present scientific tools we can neither prove nor disprove the existence of spirits of whatever nature they may be and, since we have not yet established a multidimensional paradigm that allows the inclusion of other dimensions, we have to admit our limitations. We can however, investigate what led up to such beliefs and we can evaluate results observed in the context of faith. (p. 1)

Regardless of whether these elements of psi or paranormal healing are viable methods or not, the essential healing elements (Appendix B) can be easily identified throughout the Filipino indigenous healing systems, including psychic surgery and other practices of the Filipino espiritistas. Neither the use of shamanic trickery, therapeutic sleight-of-hand, nor treatments validated by empirically based scientific research appear to be of concern to most Filipinos and many others who are open to alternative healing systems and diverse treatment modalities.

## Brody and Brody's Model

Howard Brody, M.D., Ph.D., and Daralyn Brody (2000) contend that "Twentieth-century medical science thought it had successfully banished the mind from the healing process" (p. 245). They support the "meaning model" as especially useful in organizing the large body of available information, similar to a meaning-centered model promoted by Arthur Kleinman. The attachment of meaning to illness and health is one aspect of many forms of alternative healing, which rivals the biomedical model. The psychology of healing is an area requiring further research in mainstream biomedical communities.

> If you accept the premise that the mind is not just in the brain but the mind is part of a communication network throughout the brain and body, then you can start to see how the physiology can affect mental functioning as well. (p. 87)

The "inner pharmacy" is an appropriate metaphor for the process of the placebo response, explaining the more general term of placebo effect. One of the human body's most impressive features is its ability to maintain and heal itself. When made ill by germs or disease, the body's immune system does battle and eventually (in most cases) effectively rejects or adapts to the toxins that enter the body. Brody and Brody (2000) promote viewing this human capacity as accessing the body's inner pharmacy. Environmental factors affect the way the inner pharmacy operates. Our own healing behaviors and interventions by others awaken our inner pharmacy, causing it to respond more promptly and efficiently to germs and illness. 'The metaphor sheds new light on how cures are produced by placebos" (p. 46). More research is needed in the study of neural, immune, and biochemical pathways that are affected by meaningful stimuli in human beings. "Current research into peptide receptors appears to be highly important for understanding the placebo response" (Brody, cited in Harrington 1977, p. 85).

## Kleinman's Treatment Approach

Brody and Brody (2000) and Kleinman (1988a, 1988b) promote notions of illness meanings and meaning-centered models. They are examples of what some writers call the 21st century's information based healing models (S. Krippner, personal communication, February 12, 2003). In *The Illness Narratives* (1988b) and *Patients and Healers in the Context of Culture* (1980), Kleinman developed a questionnaire for eliciting illness meanings from patients. The meaning-centered model Kleinman promotes in these books presumes that a positive placebo response is likely to occur when a treatment changes the meaning of the illness for the patient. This meaning is most likely to change when the individual has rapport with the practitioner, is listened to, and receives an explanation for the illness. The individual experiences care and concern from the healer in the healing environment. The individual feels an enhanced sense of mastery or control over the illness or the illness symptoms (Kleinman, 1980, p. 84). Kleinman's contentions are included as essential elements of healing (Appendix B) and are consistent with other systems of healing models.

Kleinman (1980) proposed a series of questions to elicit individuals' illness meanings. A determination is then made as to the participant's explanatory model or the "clinical reality" from which the model arises. These clinical realities reflect differing worldviews and very personal beliefs about the self. Some of the alternative explanations for illness in the Philippines include evil spirits, witches, engkantos (fairies) who live in the trees, or ancestral spirits. Other alternative explanations for illness could include a spell cast by a neighbor or sorcerer. After conducting an interview according to Kleinman's interview questions (see Appendix C), it should be possible to determine considerable information reflecting an individual's worldview and elicit the patient's confidence. Kleinman's questions provide a conceptual framework to gather pertinent information. This systemic cross-cultural approach began with techniques to develop trust and rapport and, subsequently, moved on to the elicitation of illness meaning (Kleinman, 1987, 175-179) and, consequently, the patient's faith and beliefs. Then one can determine a patient's optimal treatment options.

## Additional Delimitations

I was advised early in my research by Ruth-Inge Heinze, Ph.D. (personal communication, September 2, 2000), of Saybrook Graduate School and Research Center in San Francisco, that the tambalans' self-reports could not be considered reliable. "They will tell you what they think you want to hear." Heinze and others contend that the major threat to credibility is insufficient time in the field for the researcher to fully understand the lived-through experiences of the individuals and groups studied. To ensure greater reliability and a measure of conformity, the researcher must obtain more detailed evidence from informants in order to verify information across reports. Researchers must also understand the data within a holistic context, inclusive of contextual and environmental factors. Heinze and others recommend the use of triangulation of data sources to improve reliability.

I was able to implement the triangulation of data sources while interviewing the tambalans, accompanied by my wife and her relatives, who were assisting me as translators and sources of peer debriefing. My helpers were natives of the Philippine culture, lived in reasonable proximity to the tambalans who were interviewed, and were familiar with them personally and by their reputations as healers in the community. By applying triangulation of data sources, the responses of tambalans from interviews were counter-balanced for greater objectivity and credibility.

# X. SUMMARY AND CONCLUSIONS

The Philippines are a part of the world that is rich in some of the most dynamic, intense, and effective forms of health treatments that have been practiced for many centuries (Licauco, 1977, 1992, 1999; Martin, 1998; H. Martin, personal communication, November 2, 2002; McDowall, 1998). Some patients claim to have been healed of specific ailments that were not responding to conventional Western biomedical treatments. Some patients perceive their healing experiences to be nothing short of a so-called miracle or a paranormal intervention. The testimonies of these patients indicate that, perhaps, the Western biomedical model could find benefit from this ancient wisdom regarding these essential elements of healing practices.

Martin's (1998) contentions regarding the efficacy of sleight-of-hand psychic surgery refer to the role of human consciousness in illness and healing. This is consistent with Kleinman (1988a, 1988b), Frank and Frank (1991), Torrey (1986) and other proponents of the systems of healing models. is a good fit with the parameters of complementary and alternative medicine (O'Connor et al., 1997) and other systems of healing models. Western patients who have been successfully treated by these alternative practitioners have a commonality in worldview with the indigenous Filipino healers. Both groups utilize viable healing systems that exist as alternatives to the Western biomedical model.

In cultures where poverty is prominent, indigenous healing systems are available to the common people when Western biomedical care is not. Methods of mind/body medicine and other traditional healing methods often are used that utilize the essential elements of healing. In these cultures, healers "rely solely on their ability to manipulate the mind set and expectations of their patients in order to activate the healing processes that lie dormant within the patient" (Martin 1998, p. 162). In the West, we would refer to this as placebo effect/response. In underdeveloped countries, mind/body medicine is the ancient effective alternative to scientific medicine. 'The understanding of what we call hypnosis and the placebo effect may have been the basis for the development of shamanic systems of healing ritual from the earliest stages of human existence" (p. 162).

Furthermore, a Western subculture has existed with a parallel interest in alternatives to the scientific approach ever since the biomedical model emerged in the last few centuries. An explosion of interest in alternative healing systems took place from the 1960s to the 1990s and captured the interest of many curiosity seekers, psychical investigators, and patients who had been failed by the biomedical model. Many of the curious and interested who were in search of a cure traveled to the Philippines to experience the indigenous healing modalities. Accounts of personal experiences suggest that many of those who lacked faith in the biomedical model and preferred to utilize alternative or indigenous healing systems were more likely to benefit from the use of these systems.

The systems of healing models apply well to most indigenous healing systems. The essential elements of healing can be identified within most illness and healing experiences all over the world. The roles of human consciousness and meaning both play important roles in the activation both of illness and healing. The Filipino espiritistas are masters at applying the essential elements of healing within their own cultural context. Filipinos and many other indigenous peoples are likely to accept healing methods based on their faith and belief, and they respond to them positively in ways that are reported as nothing short of remarkable (Licauco, 1999; Martin, 1998, 1999; McDowall, 1998).

Although the practices of Filipino faith healing are well known, there is a great lack of information, even from the Filipinos themselves, regarding indigenous practices. Mind/body medicine is prevalent in the Philippines, and the islands offer numerous opportunities for the study of the role of human consciousness in illness and healing experiences from an indigenous perspective. The absence of quality information is due mainly to the historical suppression of indigenous healing methods by the Catholic Church and increasing industrialization and Westernization in Southeast Asia. Linguistic, cultural, and conceptual barriers increase the difficulty of gathering information and investigating the validity of indigenous healing practices. After completing this study and describing one of the indigenous healing systems practiced in the Philippines, two main reasons were identified as to why there is a lack of current information.

The first cause of the information gap is that the serious study of Filipino indigenous medicine and faith healing has been largely neglected by scientific and academic communities because the phenomenon of psychic surgery appears to defy the laws of medical science and exceeds the belief systems of most serious researchers. The most publicized investigations of the practice of psychic surgery took place from the 1960s to the 1970s, from within the narrow framework of the Western biomedical model, or were performed by psychical researchers and curiosity seeking laypersons from outside the mainstream scientific and academic communities. These written accounts were published in popular books and magazines of minimal credibility. The narrow frameworks utilized by the investigations most often resulted in one of two possible outcomes: either the psychic surgeons were miracle workers, defying the laws of science, or they were masters of sleight-of-hand and, therefore, perceived as frauds.

Secondly, the lack of serious research of Filipino indigenous healing practices has also been due to the absence of an adequate paradigm by which to examine the phenomenon, and this absence has resulted in many misconceptions. Although numerous local Filipinos and alternative-seeking Westerners continued to report positive outcomes and remarkable cures as a result of treatments from these indigenous practitioners, debunkers have persisted in their attempts to expose them as frauds and to discourage ill persons from seeking their services.

The critical attacks on the practice came from Westerners or Western-influenced Filipinos, proponents of the dominant biomedical model who perceived the practice from the biomedical perspective only.

In the late 1960s, at the same time the practice of psychic surgery was exposed to the Western world, psychologists and anthropologists were developing new systems of healing models by which to view indigenous healing practices (Frank, 1974; Siegler & Osmond, 1974; Torrey, 1986), and social medicine emerged as a formal discipline. Some anthropologists researched the indigenous healing practices in the Philippines, most notably, Richard Lieban (1967) in Cebu and Philip Singer (1990), who documented a clinical study of psychic surgery in the United States. In the last several decades, complementary and alternative medicine has become more acceptable, partly due to the many Westerners who resisted the growth of the managed care insurance industry that dominated the already limited scope of Western medical practices.

The Filipino espiritistas' therapeutic interventions are dynamic, and this quality may contribute to positive healing outcomes. They utilize many forms of healing dating back to ancient times, such as magnetic healing (or energy medicine), spirit-directed medicine (incorporating faith and belief), herbal remedies, traditional Chinese and Ayurvedic techniques, and the use of therapeutic sleight-of hand. These time-tested practices of mind/body medicine had been negated for use in Western cultures prior to any serious investigations by proponents of the biomedical model; hence, only scant information about these alternative practices is available.

Complementary and alternative medicine, systems of healing frameworks, and social medicine have become more acceptable in recent decades. Perhaps with expanding studies in energy medicine, neuropsychology, and psychoneuroimmunology, scientific communities will further investigate the alternative methods utilized by the Filipino espiritistas. New research may well expand the knowledge base regarding the human condition and, particularly, the role of psychological factors in illness and healing experiences. As the misconceptions and the stigmatization of the Filipino espiritistas are reduced through studies using new paradigms, more serious research regarding the healing methods used in the Philippines can increase, before further Westernization, industrialization, or politics rob scientists of the opportunity.

# REFERENCES

Agoncillo, T. A. (1974). *Filipino history.* Quezon City, Pl: Garotech Publishing.

Beecher, H. K. (1959). *Measurement of subjective responses.* New York: Oxford University Press.

Brody, H., & Brody, D. (2000). *The placebo response.* New York: Harper Collins.

Cagan, A. (1990). *Awakening the healer within.* New York: Simon and Schuster.

Castillo, R. (1997). *Culture and mental illness: A client centered approach.* Pacific Grove, CA: Brooks Cole Publishing.

Christopher, M. (1975). *Mediums, mystics and the occult.* New York: Thomas Crowell Company.

Frank, J. D. (1974). *Persuasion and healing: A comparative study of psychotherapy* (2nd ed.). New York: Schocken Books.

Frank, J. D., & Frank J. B. (1991). *Persuasion and healing: A comparative study of psychotherapy* (3rd ed.). Baltimore, MD: Johns Hopkins University Press.

Fuller, J. G. (1974). *Arigo: Surgeon of the rusty knife.* Devon, GB: Hart-Davis, MacGibbon Ltd.

Garcia, B. E. (1985). *The truth behind faith healing.* Cebu City, Pl: Santo Rosario Parish.

Hanscom, D. H. *Initial Decision in the Matter of Travel King, Inc., etc.* Filed in Seattle, February 28, 1975.

Hansen, G. P. (2001). *The trickster and the paranormal.* New York: Xlibris.

Harrington, A. (Ed.). (1977). *The placebo effect: An interdisciplinary exploration.* Cambridge, MA: Harvard University Press.

Heinze, **R-1.** (1991). *Shamans in the 20th Century.* Falls Village, CT: Irvington Publishers.

Heinze, **R-1.** (1997). *Trance and healing in Southeast Asia today:* (Rev. and expanded). Berkeley, CA: Independent Scholars of Asia Inc.

Hess, D. (1993). *Science in the new age: The paranormal, its defenders and debunkers, and American culture.* Madison, WS: University of Wisconsin Press.

Jilek, W.G. (1982)Altered states of consciousness in North American Indian ceremonials. *Ethos, 10,* 326-343.

Kardec, A. (1989). *The spirits' book.* Albuquerque, **NM:** Brotherhood of Life Publishing.

Kardec, A. (2000). *The gospel: Explained by the spiritist doctrine.* Philadelphia, PA: Allan Kardec Educational Society.

Kleinman, A. (1980). *Patients and healers in the context of culture: An exploration of the borderland between anthropology, medicine, and psychiatry.* Berkeley, CA: University of California Press.

Kleinman, A. (1988a). *Rethinking psychiatry: From cultural category to personal experience.* New York: The Free Press/Macmillan.

Kleinman, A. (1988b). *The illness narratives: Suffering, healing and the human condition.* New York: Basic Books.

Kleinman, A. (1995). *Writing at the margin: Discourse between anthropology and medicine.* Berkeley, CA: University of California Press.

Krippner, S. (1976). Psychic healing in the Philippines. *Journal of Humanistic Psychology, 16* (4), 3-31.

Krippner, S., & Remen, R. (2000). *Learning guide for systems of healing course #4040.* Retrieved September 9, 2000, from Saybrook Graduate School and Research Center Web site: https://www.saybrook.edu/app/lg/cr4040.asp_

Krippner, S., & Villoldo, A. (1976). *The realms of healing.* Millbrae, CA: Celestial Arts.

LaFrance, M. (1981). Observational and archival data. In L.H. Kidder (Ed.), *Research methods in social relations* (pp. 262-291). New York: Holt, Rinehart, & Winston.

Lampis, R. (1999). *Man of light: The extraordinary gifts of a great healer: Alex L. Orbito.* Zogno (BG), Italy: Aurigra Publishing.

Lewith, G. L., Jonas, W. B., & Walach, H. (Eds.). (2002). *Clinical research in complementary therapies: Principles, problems and solutions.* New York: Churchill Livingston.

Licauco, J. (1977). *Healing without medicine.* Pasig City, Pl: Anvil Publishing.

Licauco, J. (1992). *Exploring the powers of your inner mind.* Metro Manila, Pl: Inner Mind Development Institute.

Licauco, J. (1999). *The magicians of God: Faith healers in the Philippines and around the world.* Pasig City, Pl: Anvil Publishing.

Lieban, R. W. (1967). *Cebuano sorcery: Malign magic in the Philippines.* Berkeley, CA: University of California Press.

Lieban, R. W. (1981). Urban Philippine healers and their contrasting clienteles. *Culture, Medicine and Psychiatry,* 5, 217-231.

Lieban, R. W. (1996). The psychic surgeon and the schizophrenic patient: Crisis in a medicodrama. *Culture, Medicine and Psychiatry,* 20, 291-311.

Maclaine, S. (1989). *Going within: A guide for inner transformation.* New York: Bantam Books.

Martin, **H.** (Producer & Director). (1985). *Psychic surgeon of the Philippines, Rev. Alex L. Orbito* [Videotape]. Savannah, GA: Metamind.

Martin, **H.** (1998). *The secret teachings of the espiritistas.* Savanna, GA: Metamind Publications.

Martin, **H.** (1999, January). *Unraveling the enigma of psychic surgery.* Retrieved November 22, 2000, from http://www.metamind.net/enigmaipsysur.html

Martin, **H.** (2000a). *A short spiritist doctrine: The history, beliefs, and healing practices of the spiritist healers of the Philippine islands.* Savannah, GA: Metamind Publications.

Martin, **H.** (2000b). *The Christian spiritist commentaries: Awakening to the healing presence of the spirit of truth; In depth commentaries on the hidden history and ultimate purpose of the spirits of light that heal.* Savannah, GA: Metamind Publications.

Martin, **H.** (2002a). *The origins and philosophy of Filipino Christian spiritism, Parts 1, 2* & 3. Manuscript submitted for publication.

Martin, **H.** (2002b). *The gifts of the spirit: By Reverend Antonio Agpaoa, with commentary by Harvey Martin Ill.* Savannah, GA: The Church of the Living Truth.

McDowall, **D.** (1998) *Healing: Doorway to the spiritual world.* Shepparton, Australia: Cosmos Pty.

Meek, G. W. (1987). *Healers and the healing process.* Wheaton, IL: Quest Books.

Nolen, W. (1974). *Healing: A doctor in search of a miracle.* New York: Random House.

O'Connor, B., Calabrese, C., Cardena, E., Eisenberg, **D.,** Fincher, J., Hufford, **D. J.,** et al. (1997). Defining and describing complementary and alternative medicine. *Alternative Therapies in Health and Medicine, 2,* 49-57.

Office of Alternative Medicine. (1997, January). *Complementary and Alternative Medicine at the NIH.* Budget update, 3.

Ormond, R., & McGill, 0. (1959). *Into the strange unknown.* Hollywood, CA: The Esoteric Foundation.

Pelletier, K. (2000). *The best alternative medicine: What works? What does not?* New York: Simon and Shuster.

Ponopio, I. S., Cordero-MacDonald, F. V., & Raymundo, A. A. (1994). *Sociology: Focus on the Phiippines* (3rd ed.). Quezon City, **Pl:** Ken Incorporated.

Ramirez, E. V. (1995). *Touch: An alternative spiritual healing.* Cebu City, **Pl:** Lourdes Parish.

Ramirez, E. V. (1996). *Healing: A spiritual [divine] gift.* Cebu City, **Pl:** Lourdes Parish.

Rogers, C. R. (1957). The necessary and sufficient conditions of therapeutic personality change. *Journal of Consulting Psychology, 21,* 95-103.

Sherman, H. (1966). *"Wonder" healers of the Philippines.* London: Psychic Press.

Siegler, M., & Osmond, H. (1974). *Models of madness, models of medicine.* New York: Macmillan.

Singer, P. (1990). "Psychic surgery": Close observation of a popular healing practice. *Medical Anthropology Quarterly, 4,* 443-451.

Sladek, M. (1976). *Two weeks with the psychic surgeons.* Chicago, IL: Dama Press.

Stelter, A. (1976). *Psi healing.* New York: Bantam Books.

Targ, E. (2002). Research methodology for studies of prayer and distant healing. In G. Lewith, W. B. Jonas, & H. Walach (Eds.), *Clinical research in complementary therapies: Principles, problems and solutions* (pp. 325-343). New York: Churchill Livingstone.

Tiston, R. (1983). *The Tambalans of Northern Leyte.* Tacloban City, Pl: Divine Word University Publications.

Torrey, E. F. (1972). *The mind game: Witchdoctors and psychiatrists.* New York: Emerson Hall.

Torrey, E. F. (1986). *Witchdoctors and psychiatrists: The common roots of psychotherapy and its future.* Northvale, NJ: Jason Aronson.

True, G. N. (2001). *The facts about faith healing.* Retrieved September 9, 2000, from http://www.netasia.net/users/ truehealth/ Psychic%20Surgery.htm

Valentine, T. (1973). *Psychic surgery* Chicago, IL: Henry Regnery. Vergano, D. (2000). *Health: Testing surgery's placebo effect.* Retrieved November 24, 2002, from http://www.usatoday.com/ life/health/surgery/ Ihsur009.htm

Viejo, A. (2000). Trance surgery in Brazil. *Alternative Therapies in Health and Medicine 6,* 39-49.

Walsh, R. N. (1990). *The spirit of shamanism.* New York: G. P. Putnam's Sons.

Watson, L. (1974). *The Romeo error.* London: Coronet Books.

Winkelman, M. (1984). A cross-cultural study of magico-religious practitioners. In R. 1.-Heinze (Ed.), *Proceeding of the International Conference on Shamanism* (pp. 27-38). Berkeley, CA: Independent Scholars of Asia.

Winkelman, M. (1992). *Shamans, priests and witches: A cross cultural study of magico-religious practitioners.* Tempe, AZ: Arizona State University.

Wood, G. (1977). *Fundamentals of psychological research.* Boston, MA: Little, Brown.

Woodward, C. V. (1955). *American attitudes toward history.* Oxford, England: Clarendon Press.

World Health Organization. (1977). *The promotion and development of traditional medicine.* Retrieved February 15, 2003, from http://www.who.int/ medicines/library/trm/tradpromotion.shtml

World Health Organization. (2000). *The work of WHO in the Western Pacific region.* Retrieved February 15, 2003, from http://www.wpro.who.int/rd/ chapter3_4a.asp

World Health Organization. (2002). *APIAAction Plan* 2000. Retrieved February 15, 2003, from http://www.wpro.who.int/pdf/apia.pdf

Wright, D., & Wright, C. (1974, January 31). Faith or fake healing? *Woman's Home Companion,* 70-73.

# APPENDIX A

Parameters for Description of Complementary and Alternative Medicine

Lexicon:
What are the specialized terms in the system?
How are common health and illness terms distinctively defined by the system?
What are the terms used to identify roles and people within the system?

Taxonomy:
What classes of health and illness or disease does the system recognize and address?
What causes for illness does the system recognize?
How important is it to identify and address ultimate, as opposed to proximate, causes of illness?

Epistemology:
Is there a canonical body of knowledge?
How do the origins and social history of the system relate to current theories and practices?
What are the internal disputes and variables of the system? How does the system respond to novel input?

Theories (Links to Taxonomy and Epistemology):

What are important human systems, their mechanisms of action, and their interconnections understood to be?
How are the symptoms interpreted within the system, generally and specifically?
What is the relationship of preventative and therapeutic actions to illness and prevention or melioration of illness?
What is the role of patient's beliefs or expectations or practitioners' intent?

Goals for Interventions:
What are the primary goals of the system?
Outcome Measures:
What constitutes a successful intervention? How are successful interventions evaluated?
How are the successes and failures of treatments and practitioners explained?

Social Organization:
What are the prevalence and distribution of this system? Who uses the system or to whom is it particularly accessible? What is the system's referral network?
Are there specialist practitioners? What kinds of specialists are there? What are the usual therapeutic practice sites?
What are the system's internal and external legitimization and oversight structures?
What therapeutic measures are undertaken at home or elsewhere, on one's own or with the aid of family members?
How are practitioners compensated?
How does the system interact with other CAM systems?

Specific Activities and Materia Medica:
What do practitioners do?
What is the specific materia medica?
What are the classes and purposes of interventions?

Responsibilities:
What are the responsibilities of practitioners? What are the responsibilities of patients or clients?
What are the responsibilities of family or community members? Are there consensual ethical norms?

Scope:
How extensive, varied, or specialized are the system's applications?

Analysis of Benefits and Barriers:
What are the risks and costs of the system from the insider's perspective?

Accommodation and Views of Suffering and Death: How does the system view suffering and death?

Comparison and Interaction with Dominant System:
What does the system provide for healing and for coping with illness that the dominant system does not provide?
How does this system view interaction with the dominant system?
(O'Connor et al., 1997, pp. 53-56)

# APPENDIX B

Essential Healing Principles and Common Factors in Healing

|   | Shared Worldview of Healer | Personal Qualities | Patient Expectations | Techniques Procedures |   |
|---|---|---|---|---|---|
| A. Nature of the ailment | 1A | 2A | 3A | 4A | 5A |
| B. Nature of the patient | 1B | 2B | 3B | 4B | 5B |
| C. Nature of the environment | 1C | 2C | 3C | 4C | 5C |
| D. Nature of the treatment | 1D | 2D | 3D | 4D | 5D |
| E. Interactive factors | 1E | 2E | 3E | 4E | 5E |

(Krippner & Remen, 2000, p. 36)

# APPENDIX C

Kleinman's Interview Questions

What do you call the problem? What name does it have? What do you think caused the problem?
What do you think the sickness does? How does it work?
How severe is the sickness? Will it have a long or short course? What kind of treatment do you think the patient should receive? What are the important results you hope to receive from this treatment?
What are the chief problems the sickness has caused? What do you fear most about the sickness?
(Kleinman, 1988a, p. 74)

# APPENDIX D

Glossary

Definition of Terms, Abbreviations, and Conventions

CAM Parameters: The standards for inquiry and description of complementary and alternative medicine as presented by a commissioned panel to the National Institutes of Health Office of Alternative Medicine in 1995. The detailed categories of the complementary and alternative medicine (CAM) parameters provide a framework for describing systems of healing where formal theories need not be proposed. The open-ended nature of the CAM parameters makes a comprehensive qualitative inquiry possible according to varying cultural definitions.

Catharsis: An intense emotional experience that creates a feeling of emotional or spiritual release and purification. In psychology, catharsis is perceived as the process of purging, or bringing to the surface, repressed emotions in an effort to identify and relieve them.

Christian Spiritism: "An interpretation of Christian doctrine that emphasizes the role of the Holy Spirit. Spiritism in the Philippines originally derived from the amalgamation of Christianity and pre-existing shamanic and animistic beliefs. Christian Spiritism was formulated by the Filipinos along lines of the philosophy of the French spiritualist Allen Kardec." (Martin, 1998, p. 244)

Dematerialization: "The disappearance of temporarily or permanently organized substances in various degrees of solidification" (Meek, 1987, p. 61). Observers speculated that perhaps the psychic surgeons could actually perform this task, by making human tissue disappear.

Healers' Circle: Alex Orbito founded this international group of healers in 1981. This organization was formed in response to the growing international healing interests and influences of other cultures in the Philippines. Orbito accepted associate members from around the world, including Reverend Harvey Martin, who was appointed the Healers' Circle vice president for the United States.

Kardec, Allan: Norn de plume of a French Spiritualist who published *The Spirit's Book,* in 1857 near the beginning of the spiritist movement in Europe. In this book he and two mediums asked 1,018 questions of spirit entities. The spirits purportedly answered questions about life on earth and life in the spiritual world. Kardec-influenced spiritists are prevalent in Brazil and the Philippines.

Magnetic Fluid: According to *A Short Spiritist Doctrine,* magnetic fluid is a type of universal energy that comes from the earth, from minerals, from vegetables, and from animals. The animal "liquid" that emanates from the human body is curative in and of itself. "The impulsion of magnetic fluid, willed by the Holy Spirit, is directed through the body of the healer into the patient" (Martin, 1998, p. 188). The Filipino espiritistas perceive this healing energy as a liquid (see *bisa* in the translation of Visayan Cebuano and Tagalog terms section).

Magnetic Healing: "A form of healing in which the healer sends a supply of prana or magnetic energy to the affected parts of the patient, thus stimulating the cells and tissues to normal activity and ejecting waste matter from the body. This is normally accomplished by either passing or laying of hands on the affected patient. This is a universal practice that dates back to ancient history." (Licauco, 1977, p. 7)

Materialization: The alleged appearance of temporary or organized substances possessing human, animal, or mineral properties. Materialization is the act of bringing something into existence from an unknown place oforigin. For example, psychic surgeons allegedly manifest and extract tissue-like material (ectoplasm) and other substances from the human body.

Mediumship: The capacity, function, or profession of a spiritualistic medium. A person held to be a channel of communication between the earthly world and the realm of spirits, or a person with the capacity to be possessed by a spirit. In the context of Christian spiritism, it is perceived that the Holy Spirit will initiate the operation of spiritual gifts through the medium. While in trance, some mediums may speak, write, or perform healings.

Mediumship Training: With the aid of information given by a qualified instructor, the medium candidate can learn the skills to function in a deep trance. The training consists of fasting, guidance, prayer, and worship. "Such training may take many years, or a few weeks depending upon the existing predisposition of the medium." (Martin, 1998, p. 128).

NCCAM (National Center for Complementary and Alternative Medicine): Established in 1998 by a congressional mandate, the former NIHOAM office elevated its status to become an official center of the National Institutes of Health. Its purposes include training of researchers and providing public and professional information about alternative medicine.

NIHOAM (National Institutes of Health Office of Alternative Medicine): Founded in 1992, its mission was to determine priorities for the future research of complementary and alternative medicine. In 1996, it was designated by the World Health Organization as the Collaborating Center for Traditional Medicine.

Paranormal: Scientifically unexplainable phenomena relating to an order of existence beyond the visible observable universe; departing from what is usual or normal; especially so as to appear to transcend the laws of nature, often attributed to an invisible agent, such as a spirit or a ghost.

Parapsychologist: A person involved in parapsychological research, such as investigations of telepathy, clairvoyance, and psychokinesis, while also being an active member of the Parapsychological Association; exemplified in this study by Stanley Krippner.

Parapsychology: A field of study concerned with the investigation of evidence for paranormal phenomena, such as telepathy, clairvoyance, and psychokinesis. Many of the investigations of the Filipino espiritistas were performed by laypersons or psychical researchers with some background or interest in parapsychology.

Possession: It is believed that mediums call spiritual entities into their body. "The term medium is selected because they engage in some form of possession alternate state of consciousness (ASC), during which spirits are believed to take over the medium's body and operate through it" (Winkelman, 1992, p. 59).

Prana: A Sanskrit term describing the "universal force that causes matter to form bonds or to disperse. It is the vital energy that infuses all things. To possess wisdom of this vital magnetic energy is an ancient source of spiritual knowledge in nearly all cultures" (Licauco, 1977, p. 7).

Psi Healing: Psychic healing techniques are directed at affecting the human body's electromagnetic fields. These electromagnetic fields include and provide information about energy blockages and causes of illnesses. "Healing interventions can take place at this etheric level" (Stelter, 1976, p. 54). Many observers have speculated that psychic surgeons frequently perform psi healing.

Psychical Research: The research of phenomena lying outside the sphere of physical science or rational knowledge. Research which addresses the nonmaterial aspects of being, which are spiritual or beyond normal in origin. The research is sensitive to nonphysical or supernatural forces or influences, marked by extraordinary or mysterious sensitivity, perception, or understanding.

Psychic Surgery: A specialized modality or subset of spiritual healing, allegedly conducted by using the bare hands to enter the body. Espiritistas, while professing to be possessed by the Holy Spirit or other spirit entities, extract tissues, tumors, or other obstructions from the human body while the patient is conscious, without pain or the use of anesthetic, without leaving any scars, or with only minimal scaring.

Spirit Directed Medicine: The healer need not exert effort except to touch the patient or an object with the hand. Objects held by the medium can be vehicles for curing: blessed oil, water, paper, a handkerchief, and so on, all of which can cure if they have been touched by a spirit medium. "Through understanding and mastering these spiritual prerequisites as the primary means of healing, and fully integrating them into personal interaction with a patient, any and all forms of medicine can be instantly transformed into spirit-directed medicine" (Martin, 1998, pp. 141-142).

Systems of Healing: Theorists Torrey, Frank and Frank, Siegler and Osmond, Kleinman, and others have contributed to this overarching perspective of the important relationships between illness, patient, healer, and cure. The essential healing principles and common factors in healing are placed in a grid form by Krippner and Remen (2000) and are included in Appendix B.

Teleportation: "Occurs when an object, either animate or inanimate, which after apparent penetration, through matter such as buildings, often arrives at the scene of action following a seemingly instantaneous transmission or teleportation from nearby or miles away" (Meek, 1987, p. 61). This was a popular explanation when psychic surgeons would pull cotton balls, plants, hair, rope, and other objects out of human bodies.

Trickster: Hansen (2001) borrows from a cross-disciplinary approach to describe the trickster character type. "Tricksters have a number of common characteristics, and some of their most salient qualities are disruption, unrestrained sexuality, disorder, and nonconformity to the establishment. The trickster unifies major, but seemingly unrelated themes surrounding the paranormal. For instance, the paranormal is frequently connected with deception, and deceit is second nature to the trickster." (pp. 28-36) Hansen contends that the Filipino espiritistas are good examples of the trickster character type.

Union of Espiritistas of the Philippines: The Union was founded on February 19, 1905, by Juan Alvear and incorporated in 1909. The Christian spiritists were able to openly practice mediumship after approximately 300 years of suppression of their indigenous spiritual practices under Spanish colonization. However, this new form of spiritism emerged as Christian-based and was influenced by the spiritist teachings of Allen Kardec.

Witchcraft: Filipinos frequently regard witchcraft or sorcery as causes of both illness and misfortune. "Witchcraft can also be described as malign activities, including those of spirits and human beings capable of harming others through the use of supernatural power" (Lieban, 1967, p. 65). Cebuanos make a distinction between sorcerers and witches in the Visayas. In Northern Luzon, the espiritistas refer to illness as the result of witchcraft (rather than sorcery) when explaining these illnesses to Westerners.

*Translations of Visayan (Cebuano) and Tagalog Terms*

Aswang (Witch): In the Visayas, witches are perceived as inherently evil and have the capacity to alter themselves into animals or ghouls to inflict evil acts on others, both physically or through the use of malign magic.

Banal (Spiritual): The Visayan (Cebuano) translation. The majority of Filipinos are Catholic, but many also perceive active spiritual forces, not limited to the Holy Spirit, but also spirits in nature (trees, waterfalls, caves, etc.). These spiritual forces can effect daily life.

Barang: The most common form of sorcery practiced in the Visayas, the act of sending bugs or causing other foreign objects to enter the body of another person. Since it is the most common form of sorcery, it is often used as a general term for acts of sorcery.

Barrios (Neighborhoods): This word is interchangeable with *barranguy;* social and political units generally supported with strong family ties. Prior to Western influence, Filipinos lived in kinship groups. Each barrio has its own indigenous folk healers. In Cebu, the healers are referred to as Tambalans.

Biktima (Victim): The term refers to any type of victim, such as a victim of assault, an accident, and so on. In this study, the term is used in reference to victims of witchcraft or sorcery.

Bisa (Magnetic Fluid): The field of magnetic energy that surrounds all objects and beings, radiating out in all directions. It is believed that disturbances in the flow of the magnetic field may cause illness, and it becomes the healer's task to tap into the stream of magnetic energy and effect a rebalance.

Buyag: An inadvertent condition that occurs from the act of one individual paying a compliment to another. The individual receiving the compliment is most often a child. The result of the compliment is the infliction of illness or bad fate upon the receiving individual.

Buyagan: The person or spirit responsible for creating the condition of buyag.

Di-kilala (Unknown): The Visayan word used in describing "unnatural" in regards to the unnatural illness concept in this study. An unnatural illness is that which cannot be diagnosed in accordance with current biomedical standards. Patients who suffer from these illnesses are often referred to the local folk healers to receive treatment for suspected acts of witchcraft.

Enkantos (Tree Spirits): The belief in "nature spirits" is common in the Philippines. Perhaps the most common nature spirits are tree spirits who are, at times, capable of being anthropomorphized. They are often referred to as "the people in the trees" and are capable of inflicting malign magic in their spirit or anthropomorphized forms.

Espiritistas: A term of Spanish origin meaning persons who have the ability to channel spiritual energies for healing or to become possessed by spiritual entities. Espiritistas, or spiritual healers, in most classification systems are synonymous with mediums. Espiritistas often are able to perform spiritual and magnetic healing and, most notably in the Philippines, psychic surgery. "What Filipinos call faith healers and psychic surgeons may be classified as spiritual healers [espiritistas]" (Licauco, 1977, p. 15).

Hilot: An ancient form of massage, unique to the Philippines, that incorporates some principles of Ayurvedic medicine, based on knowledge of vital forces.

Kalusugan: Physical, emotional, and spiritual health. Free of negative symptoms, a desired state.

Kulam (Witchcraft): A spell or a hex sent from a sorcerer, which can manifest in illness or bad fate and can affect individuals or groups of individuals. Kulam is most often perceived as the cause of unnatural illnesses.

Lahid: A form of healing that supposedly removes or extracts foreign bodies or particles embedded in the flesh or bloodstream, allegedly caused by black magic, spells, or the machinations of evil forces. Lahid, according to occult tradition, dissolves or dismantles evil works that inflict diseases on victims. A white linen pouch, which contains grounded herb root particles, is massaged tenderly on the disease-inflicted area for approximately 20 to 40 minutes. Solid particles such as stones, broken glass, bones of fishes, and insects in whole or in parts, are common items removed or extracted. Garcia (1985) contends that "lahid therapy was an act of trickery and was a precursor to the practice of psychic surgery by Filipinos" (p. 16).

Likas (Natural): In this study, the term is used to differentiate between natural and unnatural illnesses. A natural illness is perceived as an illness that will respond well to Western medicine. Unnatural illnesses are often perceived as being inflicted by a sorcerer. These illnesses do not respond to biomedical treatment.

Mananambal (Doctor): Lieban (1967), Martin (1998), and, perhaps, most Filipinos refer to folk healers as mananambal. The word mananambal is simply translated as doctor, yet Western-trained doctors are not referred to mananambals. There appears to be no distinct difference in the practices of mananambal or tambalans on the island of Cebu.

Manghihilots: Traditional Filipino bone-setters, practitioners of Hilot massage.

Mangkukulam (Sorcerer): A sorcerer is not inherently evil, as is a witch. A sorcerer may be a folk-healer whose services are contracted by individuals to induce malign magic as a justifiable act of retribution for wrong-doing.

Nabuksan (The Opening): "Among the Filipinos, this spiritual opening, which allows someone to function in trance, is called nabuksan. The role of the mediumship trainer is to instruct, guide, and monitor the development of the medium until nabuksan takes place. In order to do this, the trainer must be endowed with special gifts of insight and discernment" (Martin, 1998, p. 128).

Panggagaway (Sorcery): Malign magic inflicted by a sorcerer. In the Philippines sorcery is frequently used as an act of retribution and considered a justifiable response to the wrongdoings of others.

Pasyente (Patient): An individual seeking treatment for an illness by folk healers, espirititistas, or practitioners of Western medicine.

Sakit (Illness): The absence of health, considered to be either from a natural or unnatural cause. Natural (diagnosable with biomedical standards) and unnatural illnesses (results of sorcery or supernatural forces) may affect groups or families, as well as individuals.

Sala (Sin): Acts of sin or a sinful lifestyle may result in the blockage of energy flow or a perversion of an individual's natural human (magnetic) energy, which may eventually result in a natural illness. Acts of sin include defiling the body, the temple of the Holy Spirit, through drinking alcohol, smoking tobacco, womanizing, gambling, or any act that separates one from God.

Tambalan (Medicine Person): The most literal translation for the word tambalan is medicine man or medicine person. The words tambalan and mananambal, both Visayan words, are interchangeable and have essentially the same meaning. Rebecca Tiston (1983), author of *The Tambalans of Northern Leyte,* and many Cebuanos refer to their local folk healers as tambalans.

*Tandock:* A form of healing practiced on the island of Mino, near the large island of Mindanao. "Tandock therapy included the making of half-inch incisions over afflicted areas of the body while a type of scope is attached and thick blood was drained out of the patient" (Garcia, 1985, p. 15).

Unless otherwise noted, all translations are my own with the assistance of my wife, Dolores Taubold.

# ABOUT THE AUTHOR

Scott Matthew Taubold, Ph, D., born in 1955, spent most of his life in a small isolated community in Northern California. After obtaining an AA degree in the early 70s in General Education, "later in life" Dr. Taubold continued his education. In 1993 Dr. Taubold moved to Hawaii where he worked as a counselor and case manager to support himself through school. In Hawaii he was exposed to a "melting pot" of cultures, people who did not respond well to conventional psychological models of treatment, but did respond positively to own their indigenous healing systems.

There was a lot of support for learning about the effectiveness of indigenous healing systems at the University of Hawaii-West Oahu where Dr. Taubold obtained his Bachelor degree in Social Science with a concentration in psychology in 1995, and in the Masters of Science in Counseling Psychology program at Chaminade University in Honolulu where Dr. Taubold obtained his Masters degree in 1997. Following his return to Northern California Dr. Taubold enrolled in a distance learning program, Saybrook University of San Francisco and obtained a Ph. D. in Humanistic Psychology in May 2003 after completing this dissertation titled.

Dr. Taubold has traveled to the Philippines in 1995, 2000, 20001, and 2003 to study the indigenous healing practices in the Philippines. Since then Dr. Taubold continues to study complimentary and alternative forms of medicine and indigenous healing systems, offers himself as a consultant on his website ww.psychicsurgery.net., and is continuing to write providing practical advice to people who are seeking alternative forms of health treatment.

www.ingramcontent.com/pod-product-compliance
Lightning Source LLC
Chambersburg PA
CBHW052029030426
42337CB00027B/4930